W9-ATP-919

THE BACK RUB BOOK

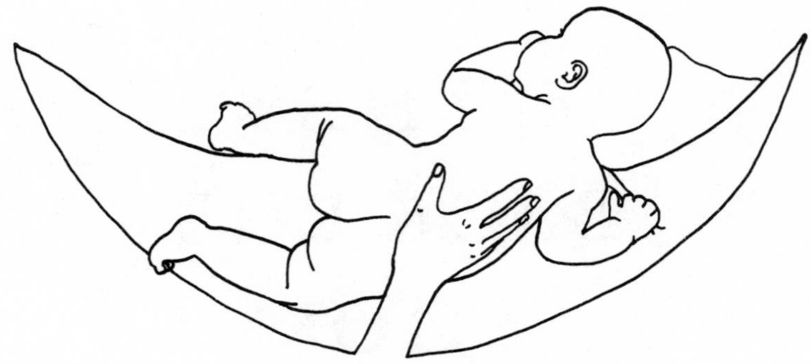

THE BACK RUB BOOK

How To Give and Receive Great Back Rubs

ANNE KENT RUSH

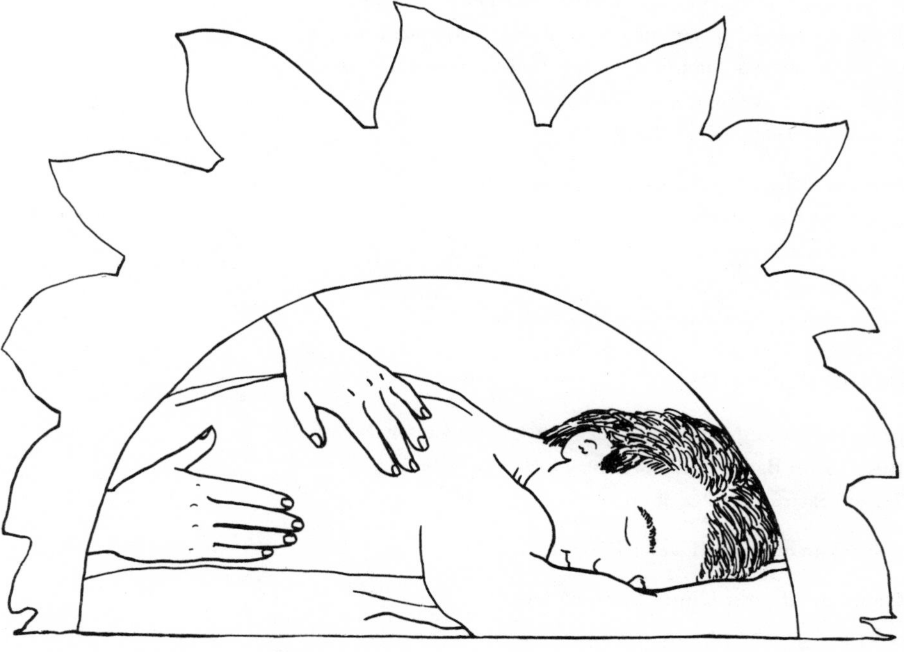

VINTAGE BOOKS A DIVISION OF RANDOM HOUSE, INC. NEW YORK

A VINTAGE ORIGINAL, JULY 1989

FIRST EDITION

 Published in the United States by Random House, Inc., New York, and simultaneously in Canada by Random House of Canada Limited, Toronto.

Library of Congress Cataloging-in-Publication Data

Rush, Anne Kent, 1945–

The back rub book.

"A Vintage original."

1. Massage. 2. Back—Care and hygiene. I. Title.

RA780.5.R87 1989 617'.560622 88-40038

ISBN 0-394-75962-1 (pbk.)

Special thanks to: Jeff Stone, Freude Bartlett, Liz Colton, Susan Sgarlat, Scott Barkdall, Bill & Donna Carey, and Dorothy & Carlos Neiderhauser-McGhee.

Book design by Maura Fadden Rosenthal

Manufactured in the United States of America

20 19 18 17 16 15 14 13

For my mother,
Cynthia Boyd Williams Rush,
who gave me my first back rub;
for Magdalene Proskauer,
whose work continues to inspire mine and
for everyone who helped—
may your lives be rich in back rubs!

CONTENTS

THE BACK RUB BOOK

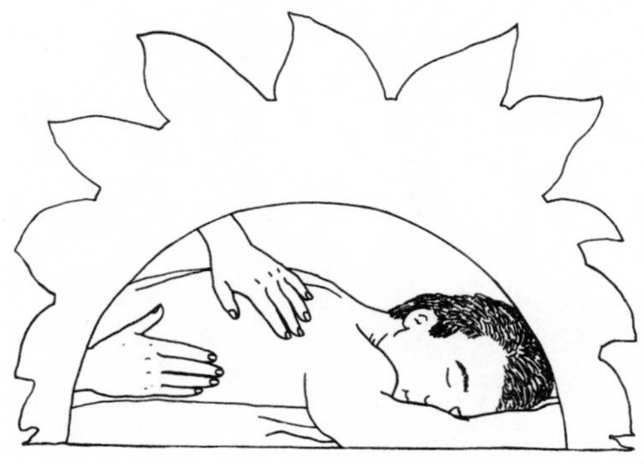

THE MAGIC WORDS

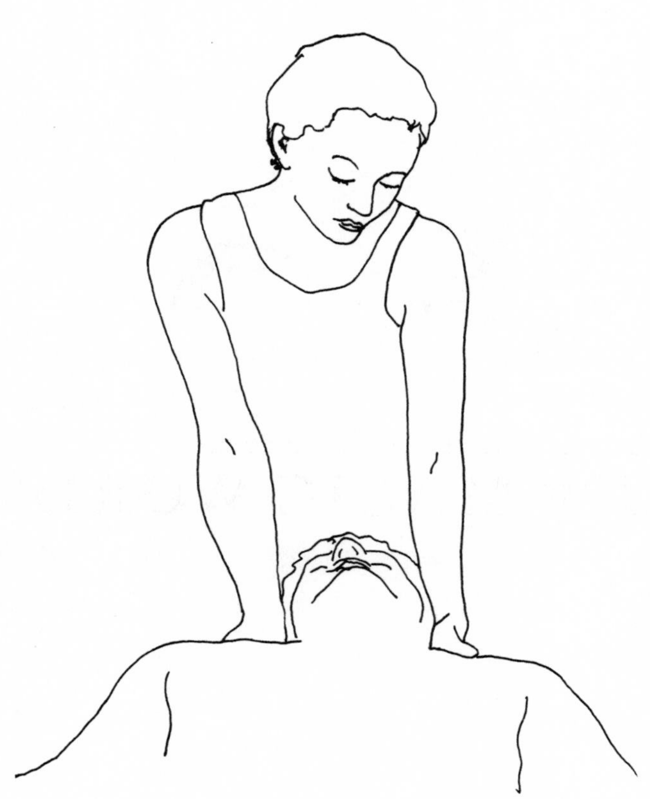

"W*ould you like a back rub?"* Who can resist this offer? A back rub is a priceless gift of caring. High on everybody's list of favorite things, a back rub refreshes you from the day's tensions. It offers a respite from physical strain, from taking care of others, and from life's stresses and responsibilities. Because many nerves radiate from your spinal cord to almost every part of the body, a back rub can ease tension throughout your whole body.

A great back rub can be done with or without oils, with clothes off or on, with your friend sitting or lying down. The bottom line to remember about back rubs is that it's nearly impossible to go wrong. People appreciate almost any kind of back rub as long as it's caring. This book can be used to enlarge and enrich your repertoire. After a little practice, you will soon be inventing your own back rubs.

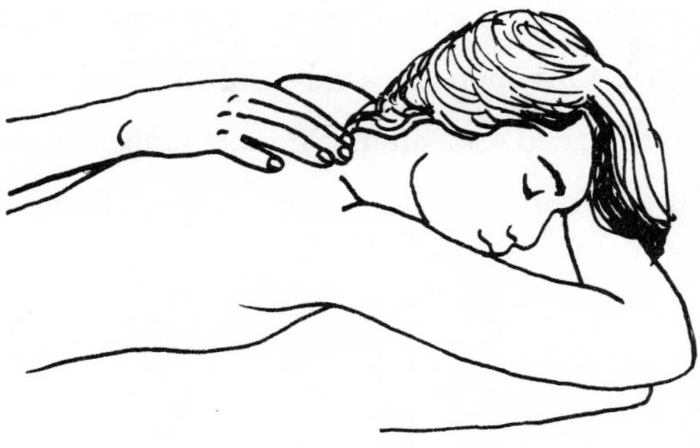

The Old-Fashioned Gift

In the old-fashioned tradition of giving handmade gifts and presents of simple caring, the back rub is tops. It is an expression of concern that comes from the heart and hands—a direct, memorable, delicious experience. A back rub gives a sense of being taken care of that money can't buy. Instead of a promise or a token, you give relaxation itself. A back rub gets right down to the basics of gift giving because a back rub is the most important of all gifts—a gift of yourself!

For a friend, back rubs are a pleasant exchange of support and sensitivity. For a lover, back rubs are an especially sensual treat. For a child, a spouse, a parent, or a grandparent, back rubs can become a family tradition imparting security and warmth.

You can tailor back rubs to fit the mood and situation so that they become the perfectly appropriate present for a variety of occasions. As an expression of thoughtfulness a back rub is the perfect gift for the person who has everything!

Like kisses and compliments, one back rub just naturally inspires another. You rarely have to ask. Give more back rubs and you're likely to find yourself on the receiving end soon after. For more relaxation, health and warmth in your life, remember the Open Sesame: "*Would you like a back rub?*"

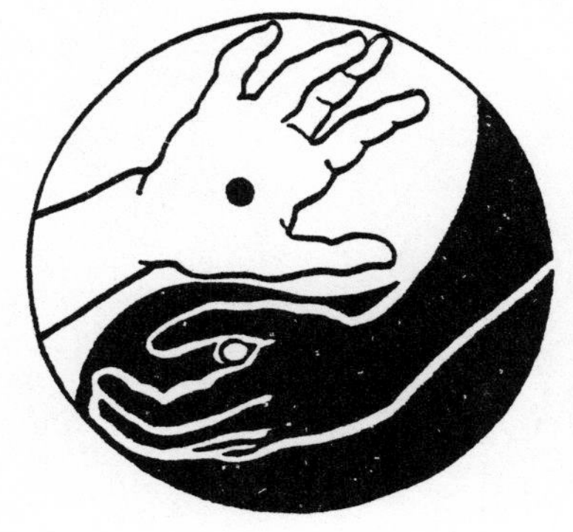

GIVING & RECEIVING

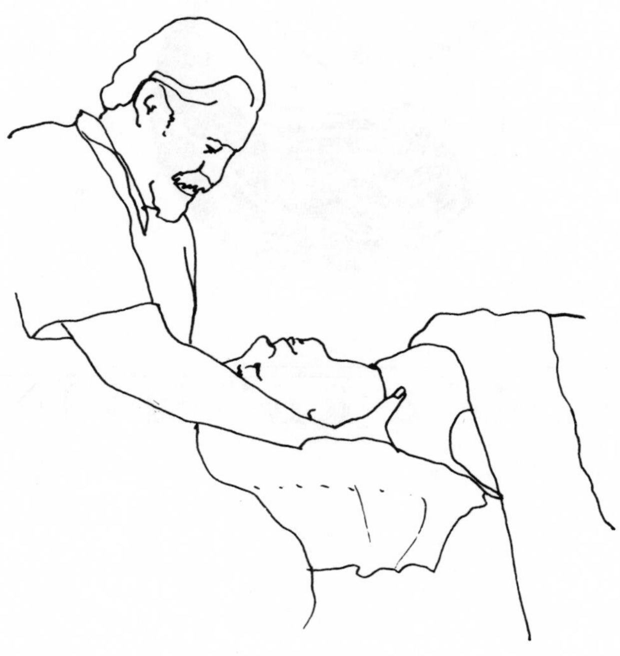

GETTING COMFORTABLE

Everybody has an idea of what makes them feel happy and at ease. If you are close to the person you are massaging, you probably know what they enjoy. If not, talk it over. The best back rubs occur when both of you are comfortable.

To Be Clothed or Not to Be Clothed?

To be clothed or not to be clothed? That is the question on the minds of most people about to be massaged. If you are giving a back rub to a veteran, she or he will probably want to shed their clothes and relax. Some people only feel comfortable when wrapped in a towel, or wearing a swimsuit, or perhaps only when fully clothed. In the latter case, use the clothing for the sliding effect that oil would have provided.

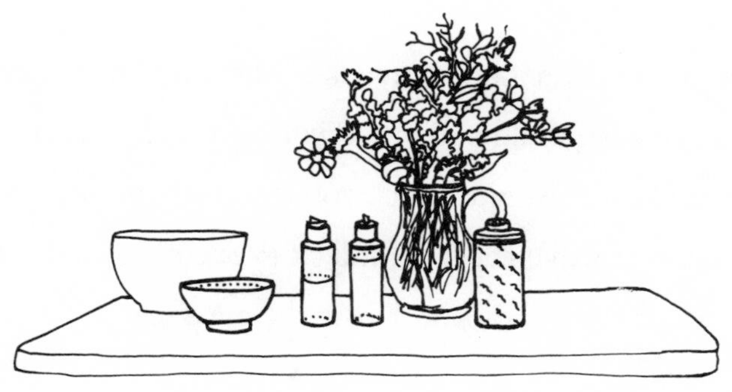

Oils

Being anointed with oils has always been considered a great honor and a luxury. In massage, the use of oils allows a thorough and sensuous treatment. You can perform a wider variety of strokes—sliding across the skin and creating continuous, smooth pressure over the muscles.

Hand lotions and baby oil are not recommended as massage oils because they are absorbed quickly into the skin. You want a lubricant that keeps on lubricating. Rubbing vegetable oil into your skin adds nutrients as well as moisture. Certain oils smell good and treat your olfactory sense during the massage.

You can mix massage oils yourself by combining any vegetable oil with an oil scent essence. Some delicious and easy preparations are described in the "Oils, Herbs and Exotics" chapter. Or you can buy massage oils at health food stores.

An oil massage takes longer than a massage without oil. You need to arrange a place with a sheet or towel to lie on. And your friend will probably want to shower afterward to prevent any oil stains on clothes.

The most convenient container for massage oils is a plastic squeeze-top bottle that you can easily hold and move with you while massaging. Pouring the oil into a small bowl into which you can dip your fingertips will also work. The drawback is that the bowl will sit in one place and may end up out of your reach at some moment during the massage.

Be sure the oil is body temperature when you apply it. Having cold oil spread on your body is the opposite of relaxing. Rubbing your oiled hands together several times before applying it will warm the oil.

Powders

Some people prefer powder as a massage lubricant. Look in a health food store or drugstore to find a powder that contains healthy ingredients. Powders made for babies often contain the best ingredients. Talcum tends to clog pores, so look for a clay base powder. Sprinkle it on your friend's back right from the shaker. You'll probably need to apply powder more often than oil for the same degree of lubrication.

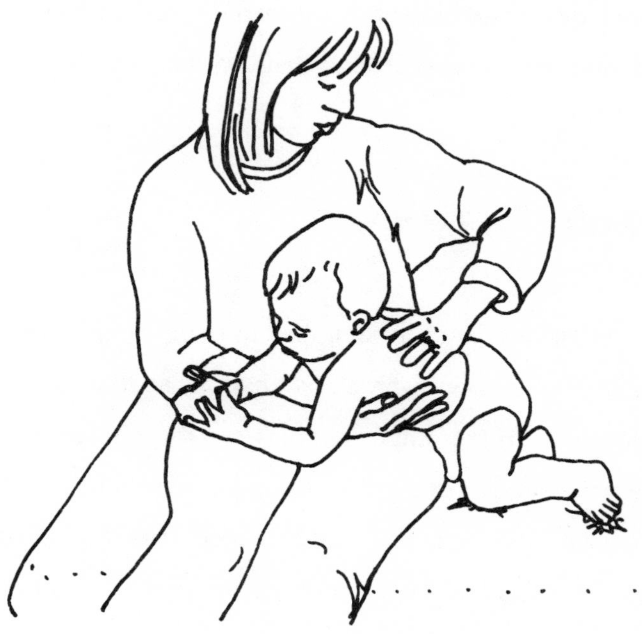

THE TICKLES

People prone to the tickles fall into four categories, with great variation in the degree of severity of affliction.

First-Degree Ticklee

First-degree ticklees are occasionally and rather unexplainedly ticklish. This category embraces a large number of people. Most of us have our ticklish moments. If you, the ticklee, are being massaged, call for oil or powder. Usually a lubricant removes slight ticklish tendencies by reducing friction. If you are giving the massage, press harder than usual. Deeper pressure tends to surmount the tickles. First-degree ticklees are usually only ticklish on their feet and around their waists.

Second-Degree Ticklee

Second-degree ticklees are self-identified as being ticklish and are quite articulate and specific about where and under what conditions they succumb. A climate of trust is important between the masseur and the second-degree ticklee to achieve a calm massage. The ticklee will tell you where the ticklish spots are. You should respect these forbidden zones so the receiver can relax. You might massage this person through a towel or sheet to reduce tickling. Use firm pressure.

Third-Degree Ticklee

The third-degree ticklee takes no prisoners. Here is a true challenge to your skill and ingenuity. Can you give such a highly ticklish, massage-resistant individual a great back rub with a minimum of feverish interruptions?

Have the third-degree ticklee sit up and rest their head on a table or sofa back while receiving a back rub. Lying down escalates the third-degree ticklee's fear of being touched in the wrong place and being undefended. Shiatsu techniques hold the most hope because pressure point massage is firm and not feathery (see page 127). If the third-degree ticklee still giggles, don't try, try again. Give up and take your friend out to dinner.

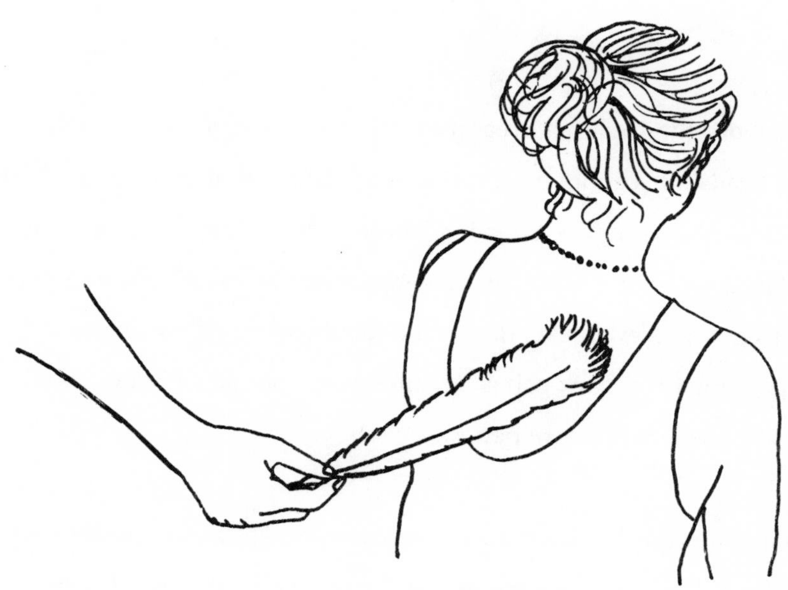

The Tickle Addict

Tickle addicts are mavericks: they love tickling more than any other skin contact. Light, feathery strokes send them into an alpha state. Stroking—without oils or any lubricant, directly on the skin—that would drive most other ticklees to reveal all their family secrets sends addicts into calm, endorphic rapture. For the most appreciated results, use your fingernails or fingertips to make repetitive, sweeping patterns on your friend's back. To present the tickle addict with a very special treat, give him or her a back rub with feathers.

TIMING

Brevity is not the soul of a great massage. However, if there is only a short time available, a short back rub is much better than none at all. Most people feel it's always a good time for a back rub—while traveling on a crowded airplane, after a hard day at work, before a marathon or a presentation, during a holiday weekend with the family, while falling asleep or waking up. Time for a back rub is any time some physical caring would help you and your friends fare better.

The back rubs in this book are relatively short, except for the unhurried Valentine Back Rub. Brief back rubs can be quite effective at relieving tension and aches. Many people who wouldn't or couldn't take more time are willing to interrupt their routines for 10 minutes of relaxation.

If possible, the longer the back rub the better. I've designed the various back rubs in this book so that each focuses on a different area of the back or on a different method. When you have a long time available, you can string several short massages together into one long back rub. If you don't know many strokes and want to do a long massage by repeating a few strokes several times, do it. A repeat performance of a good thing is often as pleasurable a treat as a new show.

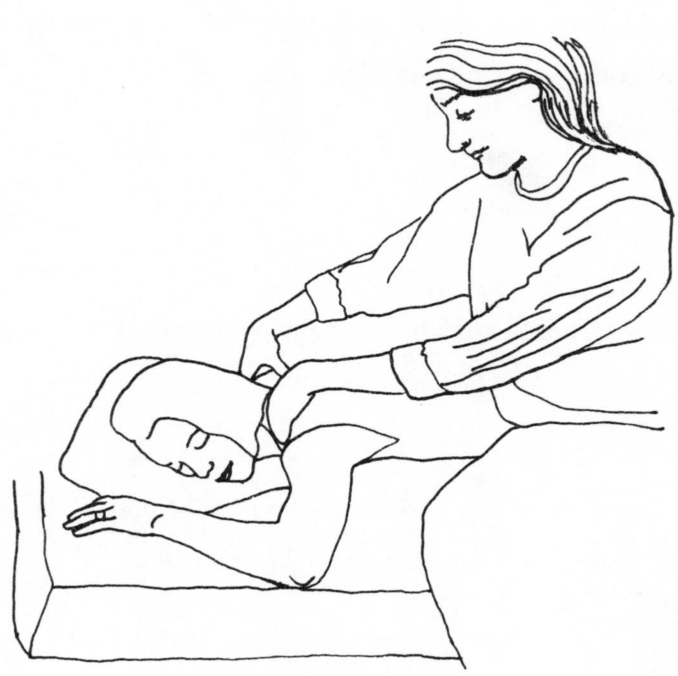

GIVING

Giving and receiving are two sides of the same skill: taking care of someone. Both are equally useful to cultivate. In massage, giving a good back rub involves refining your intuition and enjoying someone else's pleasure. Receiving a back rub involves the ability to put yourself at ease and to comfortably make your needs known.

Being skilled in only one of these personal arts soon becomes tiresome. Most people are strained by always taking the same role. Best to alternate giving with receiving. The guidelines provided here will increase your enjoyment of both giving and receiving.

Be Prepared

Here are some technical aspects that heighten the pleasure of a good massage.

Arrange a place for the massage where you will be undisturbed. Make it comfortable, warm, well ventilated, dimly lit, and quiet.

Have the oil or powder ready. Make sure it is at room temperature or very slightly warmed.

Plan your strokes beforehand so your friend doesn't have to wait while you think what to do next. Offer the opportunity to tell you what they like, where they like it, and how they like it. Some people enjoy telling you. Other people experience giving instructions as a burden. They prefer surprises.

Relax thyself, so you don't pass tension on to your friend. Allow your full attention to go toward the comfort of the person being massaged. Center yourself. (See the Basic Breath exercise on page 117.)

Have a sheet or beach towel on hand to cover your friend in case of cold. Oils tend to lower a person's temperature.

Check your hands. Be sure your fingernails are very short, your hands clean, your clothing comfortable. Remove all watches and jewelry, because they scratch.

Maintaining the Comfort

Talk as little as possible. You want your friend to be able to relax and float into her or his own reverie. Before you start, ask if there are areas to be focused on or avoided. Tell your friends you'd like to know during the massage if they want the pressure of a stroke increased or lightened. Then allow most of the communication to be nonverbal.

Use your hands to communicate relaxation to a tense muscle. Resist telling your friend that he or she is too tense. Being told to relax is usually annoying.

Keep tuned to how you are sitting, standing or kneeling so you're sure to remain comfortable yourself. When standing, bend your knees slightly to relieve back fatigue. When sitting or kneeling, try to keep your back straight and shift your weight occasionally to prevent stiffness.

Avoid developing fixed ideas about how people relax. If you're comfortable with a request, respect it. Don't insist that "relaxation" be done your way. Familiarize yourself with various methods so you can respond to different needs and tastes.

Talking and Listening with Your Hands

An essential source of relaxation in a good massage comes from not having to explain and communicate verbally. You are giving a back rub to a person as well as to a back, so each experience will be different. When you are first learning to massage, you'll need to ask for verbal feedback. As you become more skilled and comfortable, the information you need will come to you through your hands.

Relax your hands. Keep your arms and hands relaxed and learn to achieve deep pressure by leaning. Apply your body weight down your arms rather than tensing your arm muscles for pressure. This method will keep your hands from tiring quickly. The massage will also feel more relaxed to the receiver.

Move smoothly and rhythmically. Random stroking is not relaxing. Begin slowly and gently, working up to speedier rhythms and deeper pressure. Then gradually slow down and lighten up toward the end of the massage. The warm-up phase allows your friend a moment to relax and become used to being touched. The cool-down phase slows the circulation and allows your friend to relax more deeply. And it keeps the loss of physical contact at the end of the massage from being too abrupt.

Synchronize your breathing with your movements. Also try synchronizing your breathing and your movements with your friend's breathing. Make the transitions between strokes gradual and treat them as parts of

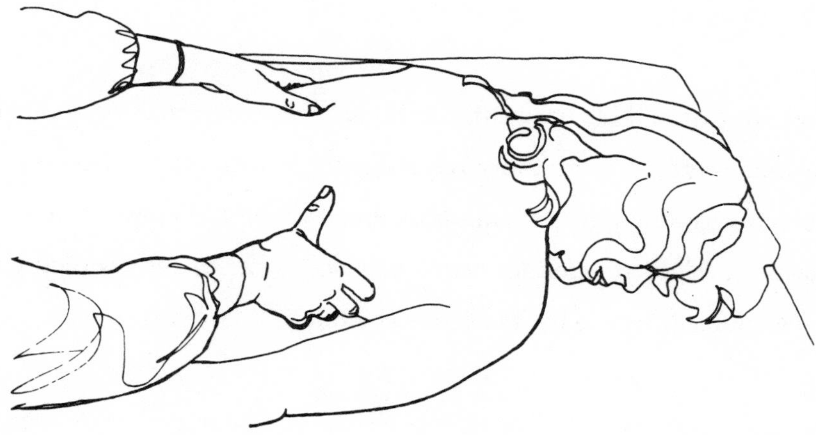

the massage. Keep contact until the end of the massage, even when reaching for oil. Discontinue anything that hurts you or your friend. Many people enjoy deep pressure, but not to the point of pain or injury. Pain makes the muscles tense and counteracts the goals of your massage.

Define the contours and deeper structures of the body you are massaging. Allow your hands to shape themselves around the bones and muscles. Part of the satisfaction of being touched is to experience one's own physical definition. The back especially lends itself to this sensation. It is a part of ourselves we normally do not see, and there is thus a special pleasure in learning about it through touch.

RECEIVING

It's your turn. This back rub is for you. Take the rare opportunity to be "self-centered." The more relaxed and comfortable you become, the more gratified the person massaging you will feel about their massage. Allow yourself to forget your daily worries and distractions. Give yourself over to the pleasures at hand.

Set the stage to suit your tastes. Before you begin, tell your friend if you have preferences about clothes or covers, kinds of oil, depth of pressure, areas to spend extra time on, areas to avoid. Speak up with any special requests.

The one person I've met who prefers giving to receiving massages says it's because he's afraid his partner will be hurt by his requests to change aspects of her massage. This kind of communication gap should not stand between you and a good massage. If this is a sore point, you can learn to present your requests as friendly information, not criticism. Explain that it's fun for you to be able to tailor the conditions, and ask for changes with affection.

Talk as little as possible. This is your chance to forget about the outside world, to forget about entertaining someone else, to relax with your own thoughts and sensations. You can increase the depth of your relaxation during the massage by focusing your attention on your friend's touch and on your physical responses. Focus on the realm of touch during the massage to complete your vacation from the rest of the world.

Your breathing can take you deeper into relaxation. Close your eyes and allow your breathing to slow down and to flow deeper into

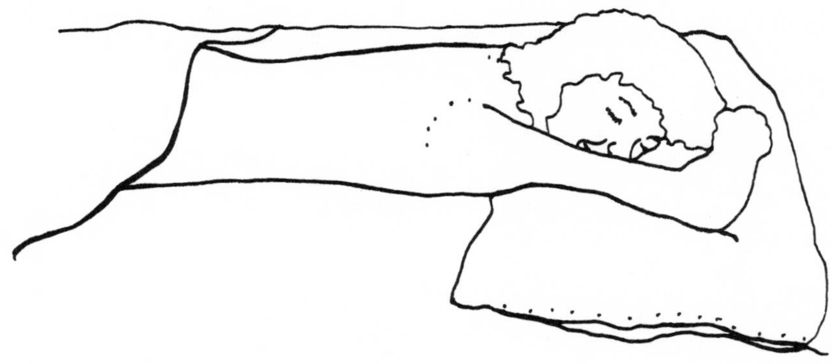

your body. Don't force a rhythm. Imagine that you can exhale downward through your body and that your breath follows your friend's touch.

At the close of the massage, allow yourself to lie still awhile. Appreciate the effects before rising.

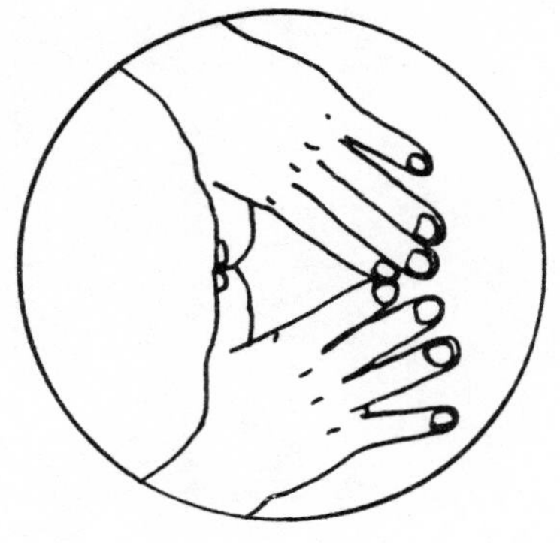

GOOD MORNING & GOOD DAY

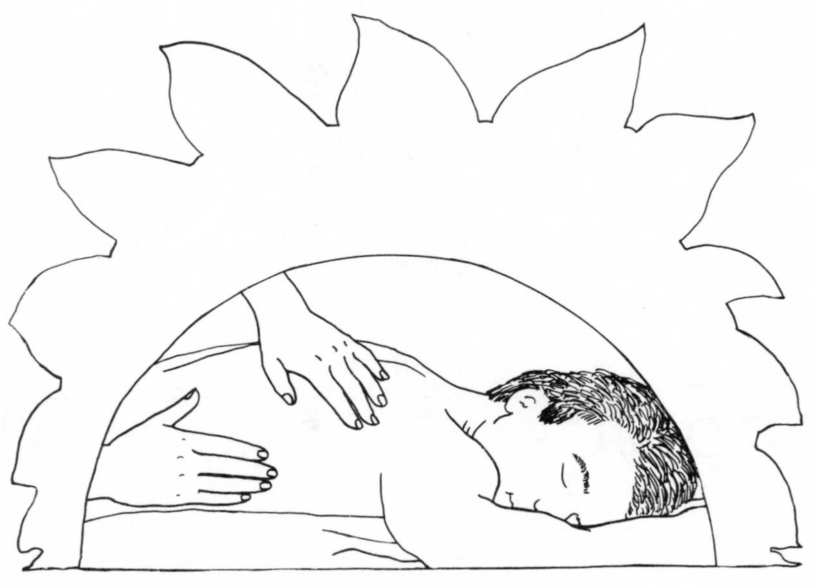

WAKE-UPS

Imagine waking in the morning and receiving a gentle, soothing back rub. What a healthy way to start the day. Your body is eased into wakefulness and your circulation is stimulated before you get up. If you plan to do exercises before starting your outside day, the good morning massage will warm up your muscles for the stretching.

Sleep to me is one of life's great pleasures. Getting out of bed in the morning is one of life's difficulties. A wake-up back rub is a gentle alarm clock that makes me glad it's morning. If you are lucky and relish rising early, a good morning back rub can be effective preventive medicine for the day's tensions.

Touching grounds you. You feel a basic relaxation all day long that comes from the morning massage. If you live with someone, the two of you can alternate days of having the pleasure of "going first." It's a great luxury to be slowly drawn into a waking state from sleep by the massage of your friend.

If you live alone, you can do the back stretches described in the work and travel section to relax your back for the day.

When you're tense, your body forgets what it is to feel good. A back rub to start the day reminds you of your most comfortable state. It offers you a guideline—a point of relaxation to return to throughout the day. Monday morning will never be the same!

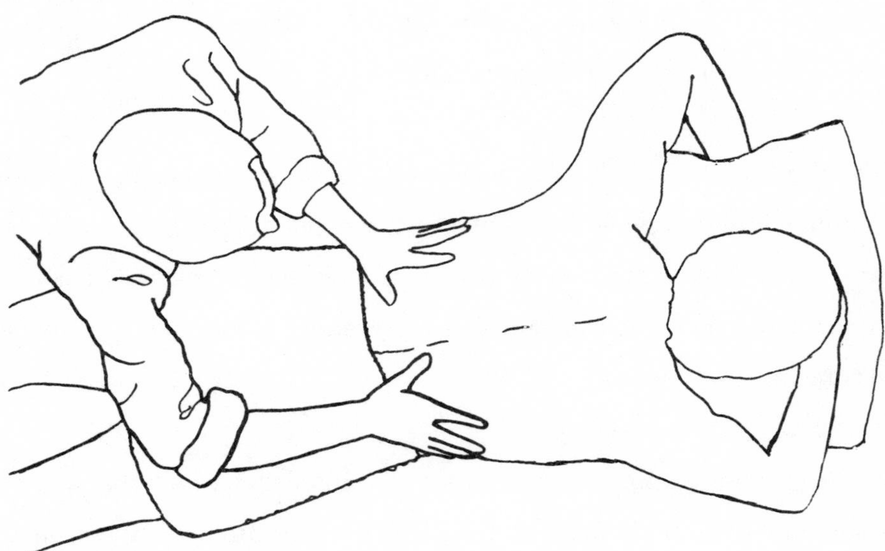

A Good Morning Back Rub

10 minutes

Upper Back Circles—4 sets
Braiding—2
Trapezius Squeeze—8
Thumb Slide—8 on each side
Palm Slides—2 down & up
Hacking—2 down & up
Patting
Braiding—1 up & down
Spine Sweep—4

A GOOD MORNING BACK RUB

The technique, rhythm and strokes of a good morning back rub are oriented to gradually speeding up the circulation, rather than slowing it down as most relaxation rubs do. It's best if this massage is short so it does not make the receiver sleepy again.

Upper Back Circles

Place your palms on your friend's back and make large, slow circles to ease them awake.

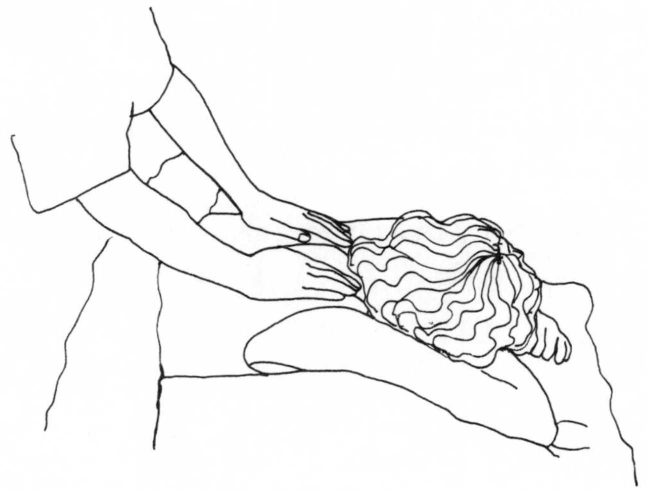

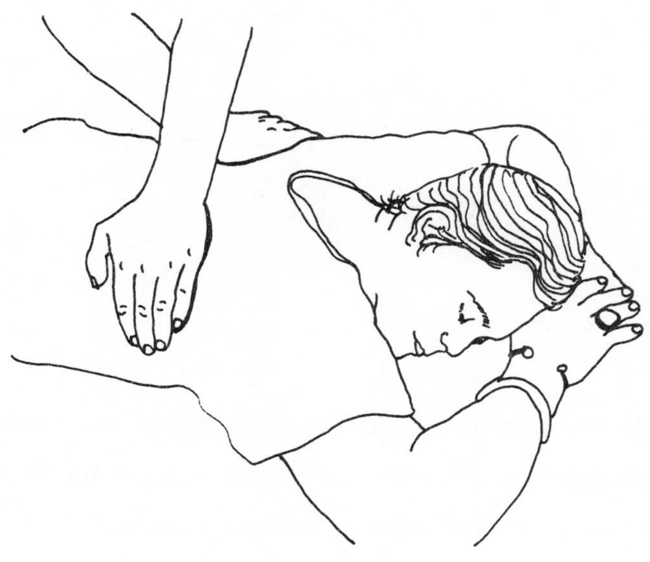

Braiding

Place your right hand on your friend's right shoulder and your left hand on his or her left shoulder. The fingers of both your hands point toward the bed. Slowly pull and press both hands, heels first, toward the spine. When the hands are about to meet, swing each hand around so that the fingers point toward each other. Moving at the same pace, press your left hand to your friend's right side and your right hand to the left side. Your forearms will form an X as your hands pass over the spine.

Your fingertips will reach the bed. Drawing your hands a little farther down the back, begin the crossing sequence again. Make your way down and up the back in a smooth, continuous motion. Start with a very slow rhythm and gradually speed up.

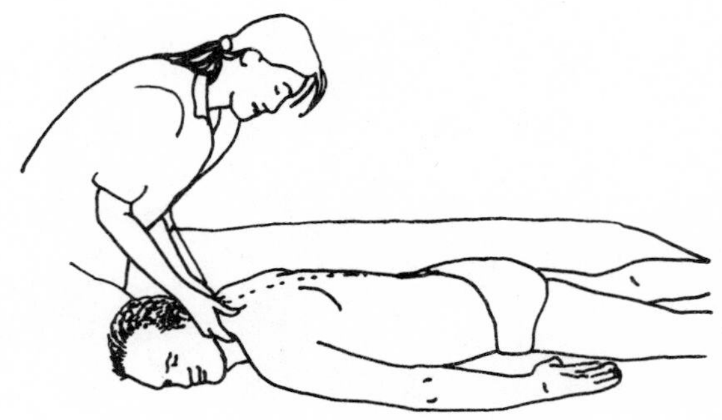

Trapezius Squeeze

On the upper back, knead the muscles curving from your friend's neck onto his or her shoulders. Working the muscles between the thumb and fingers of each hand, do both sides at once. Start with light, slow squeezes and gradually speed up and squeeze harder.

Thumb Slide

Standing to their side or above your friend's head, press and slide your thumbs away from you in short, alternating strokes. Keep your palms off the back. Stay off the bones of the spine and the shoulder blades. Massage the muscles just above the blades and those lying between the blades and the spine firmly and smoothly in a pattern like a crescent moon.

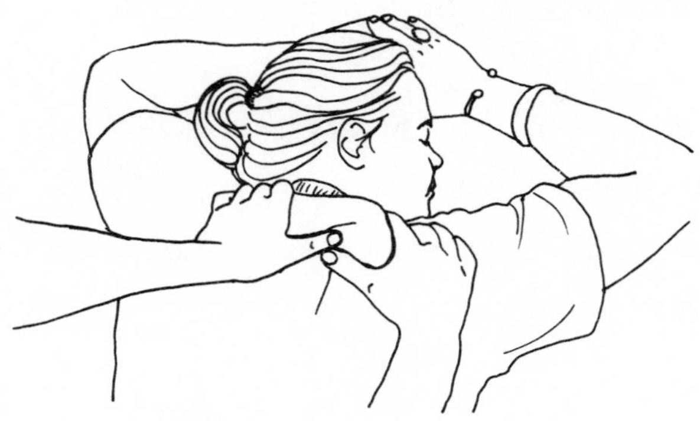

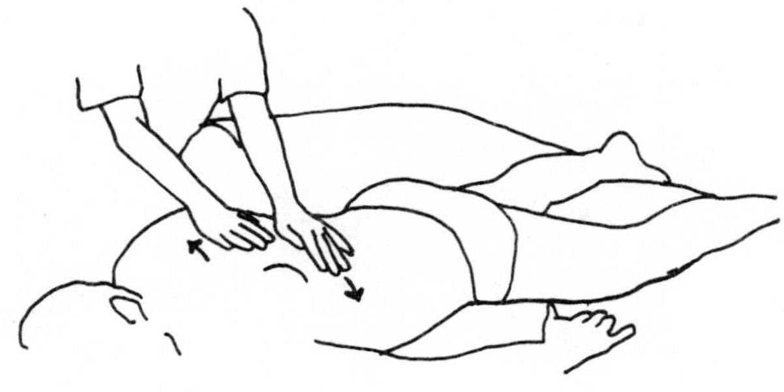

Palm Slides

Slide your palms in horizontal lines across the back. Drag your right hand toward yourself as you push your left hand away and vice versa. Without leaving the surface of the skin, keep your hands moving constantly and rapidly. Stay off the sides of the torso.

Hacking

Drum the padded outer edges of your hands lightly and very rapidly against the spine. Start at the top of the spine and work down. Next work back to the base of the neck. Then cover the rest of the back muscles.

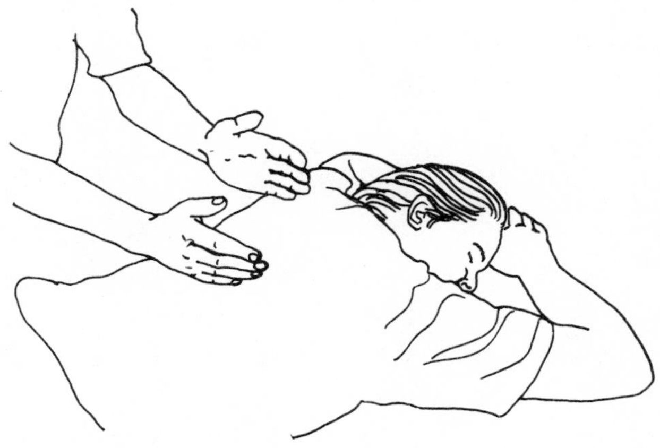

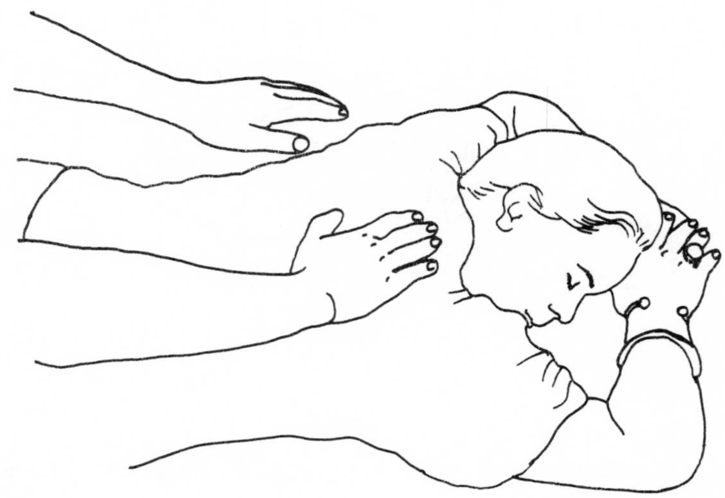

Patting

Sit to one side of your friend. Using your palms and alternating hands, simply pat your friend on the back. The secret to making this a very enjoyable stroke to receive is to set up a continuous rhythm and to keep the pressure relatively light but to use your whole palm. The pats should make a muffled clap sound. Work carefully from the shoulder of the far side of your friend's back down to the hips, then up the near side to the shoulders. Continue without a break down the far side again so the patting is performed in a circular route. End on the shoulders.

Braiding

Repeat the Braiding stroke once down the back.

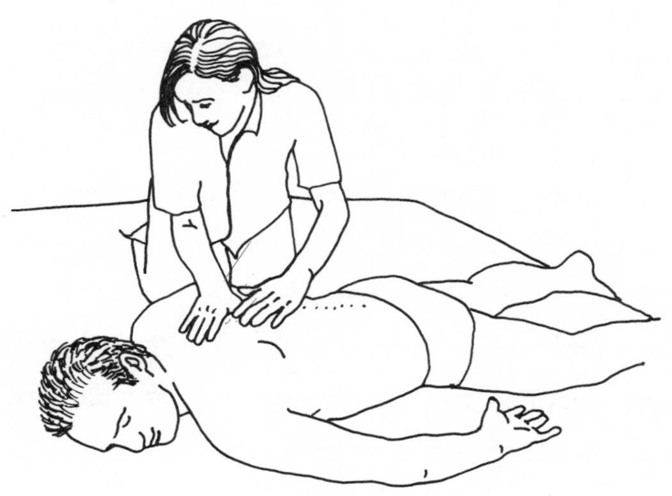

Spine Sweep

Place your palms on your friend's shoulders. Draw your hands along the muscles on either side of the spine, down the back and over the hips. As you cross the hips, angle your hands away from each other and lift them off the body. Return your palms to the shoulders and begin the sweep again with light, swift strokes.

WORKING AND TRAVELING BACKS

Most jobs put a great deal of strain on workers' backs. Back problems strike about 90 percent of people in the U.S. today and are responsible for 40 percent of all absences from work.

Executive Backs & Other Sit Downs

Muscles lose their elasticity and become prone to injury from long hours of sitting in one position. Extended plane flights and car trips are quite hard on the back. Holding the phone to one side of your neck continually can cause upper back problems. Being stationary for long periods and then suddenly engaging in vigorous, quick movements—such as lifting suitcases or boxes or playing sports after work—often injures the back. Truck drivers and machine operators have back-damaging jobs, as do writers.

Massage in the Workplace

Although massage on the job is still rare, an increasing number of companies are allowing massage office calls. Many corporations also buy and use exercise videos and send employees to back treatment classes. Some simple, effective movements and exercises you can do on the job to take care of your back follow.

Between Innings Stretches

Taking breaks, changing positions frequently, improving circulation, and releasing pressure on your back by getting up from your car or computer and walking around—these all help to save your back from injury. Sit in a chair no longer than twenty minutes. Then get up and move around awhile. Drive no longer than one hour without stopping to get out and stretch.

You can do exercises in your office or on plane or car trips several times during the day. Your back is damaged by uninterrupted, same position activity. Prevent minor tensions from snowballing. Melt them as they arise. Don't wait till they're too big to dissolve.

You can choose several of the exercises in this section to sprinkle through your day. Severe physical problems are caused by seemingly tiny stresses that occur over and over again. Brief but frequent exercise breaks neutralize this stress buildup.

Beware of the "weekend warrior" syndrome. Many workers, sedentary during the week, plunge into intense bouts of home improvement or sports on weekends that injure their out-of-shape back muscles. Moderation is the path to back health.

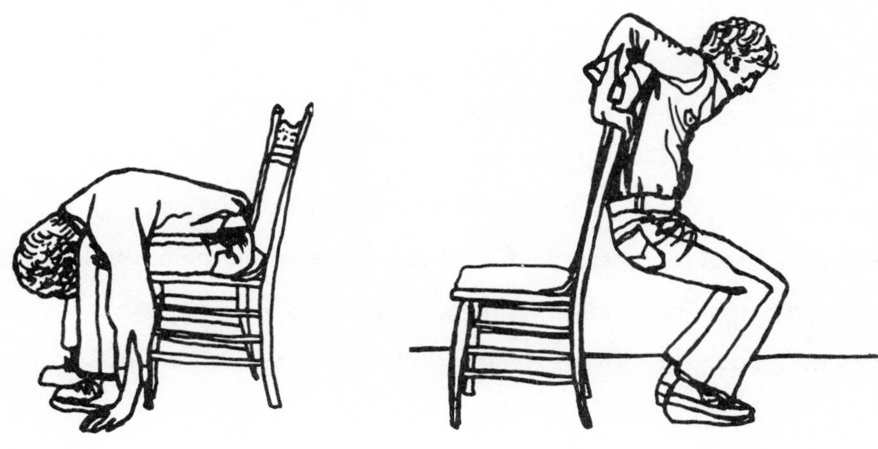

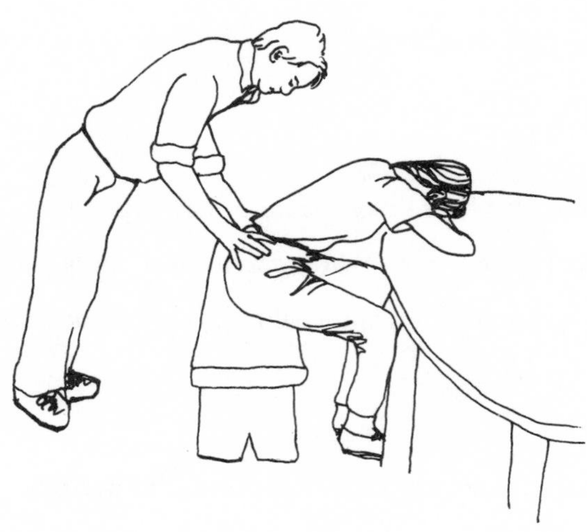

Lower Back Press for Two

If you are receiving, sit on a bench or turn a chair so the chair back is to one side and your friend can reach your lower back. Rest your head on your desk. If you are giving the massage, lodge your elbows into your ribs or above your hipbones and, leaning your weight into your arms, press with your thumbs or knuckles on your friend's lower back to either side of the spine. Lean back a bit to release the pressure and move your hands to the next area on the lower back. Apply pressure gradually with thumbs or knuckles on various spots on the sacrum and lower back.

Phone Muscle Massage

If you are receiving, lean your head on your arms on the desk. If you are giving the massage, stand behind your friend and use your hands like pincers to squeeze the muscles to either side of the neck across the shoulders.

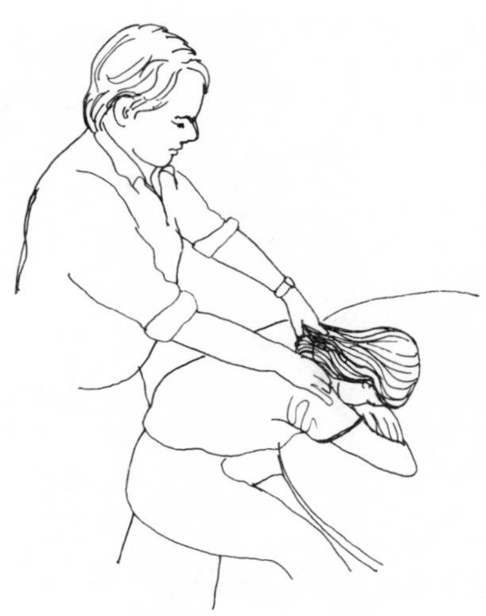

What makes this squeezing feel good is to apply and release pressure gradually, to cover the trapezius muscles thoroughly, and to work steadily and rhythmically. You can also lean your elbows gradually into your friend's shoulder muscles as he or she sits straight, and rest there as long as it is comfortable. Release gradually.

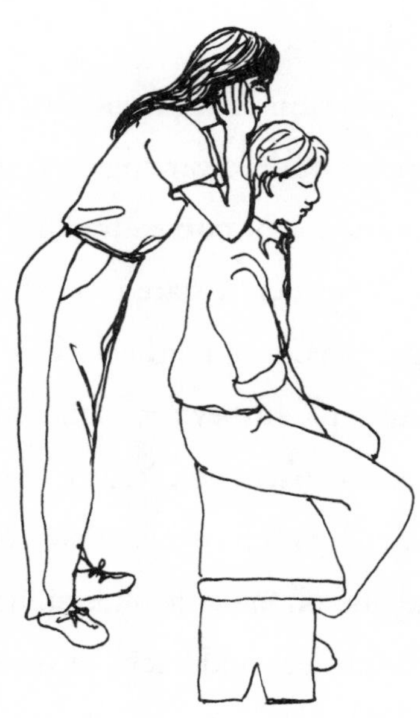

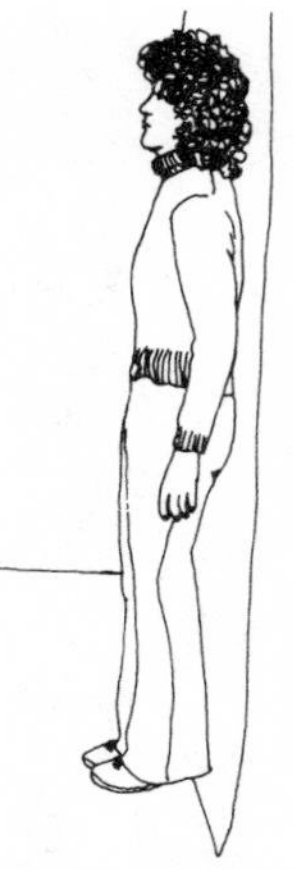

Wall Press

Great to do if you're alone in your office, this standing exercise is a variation of lower back exercises done lying down. Lean your heels, your buttocks, your shoulders, and your head against a wall. Then press your whole spine, from your lower back to your neck, backward. Try to flatten yourself against the wall. Press as you exhale. Inhale when you release.

Chair Checkup

Be sure your chair supports your lower back. Try placing a small pillow at your lower back to support your lower spine as you sit. Don't use chairs that are perfectly straight backed or curved forward at the shoulders; they encourage you to slump. Armrests that are too high and chair legs that are too low (as in theaters) strain your upper back. Use cushions to keep your knees fairly even with your hips. If they are higher or lower, the resulting pressure causes cramps and swollen feet. Your feet should touch the floor to prevent pressure on your legs. Have a rocking chair as an alternate office chair. You can read and phone in it while shifting your position and varying the pressures on your legs and back. Most important, get up and walk around quite often while working.

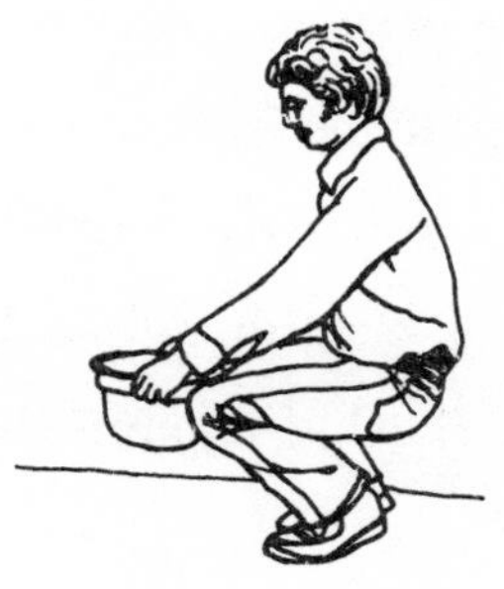

Lifting and Labor

Any heavy lifting should be done with slight flexion of the hips and considerable flexion of the knees, so that you lift mainly with the muscles in your thighs and legs rather than with the muscles in your back. Keep your elbows slightly bent and your pelvis tucked under. The best way to lift an object from the floor is to squat all the way down and pick it up while squatting. Stand up, using your leg muscles to do the lifting. Don't arch your back; keep the lumbar region around your waist straight when you squat. Keep one foot flat on the floor at all times. Hold heavy objects close to your body. Avoid lifting heavy objects above waist height. Avoid sudden movements; learn to move smoothly. Change positions frequently; this keeps you from getting cramps and maintains your flexibility.

Torso Hang

To relieve strain on your whole back, try this exercise often during your workday. Stand up. Spread your feet about hip width apart. Relax your

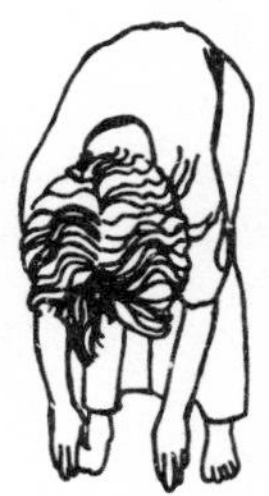

head and neck forward. Slowly, vertebra by vertebra, curl your spine forward so that your arms are relaxed in front of you toward the floor. Keep your knees slightly bent. Try to touch the floor with your fingertips, but don't strain. Don't stretch, pull, or push. Allow your arms to swing gently as you hang to loosen your back while you breathe.

Upper Back Opener

This is a great release for upper back and shoulder muscles. Stand with one foot about 12 inches in front of you, your hands clasped behind you. Keep your rear leg straight. Inhale. Bend the forward leg at the knee and lean your head and torso over that knee. As you lean raise your arms behind you. Stretch your arms so you can feel your shoulder pockets open and your shoulder blades move toward each other. Exhale as you lower your arms and stand up straight again. Repeat this motion bending your other leg.

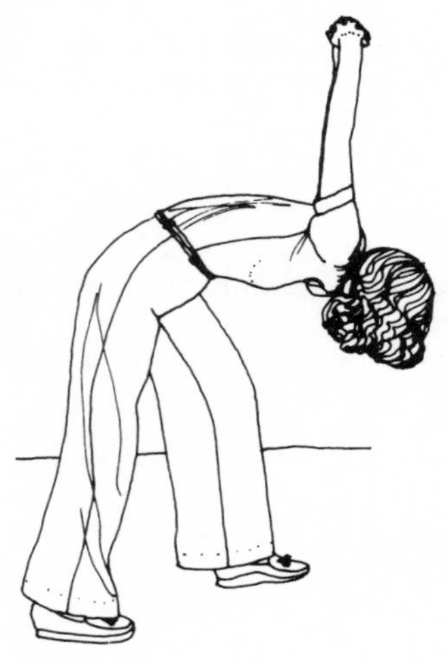

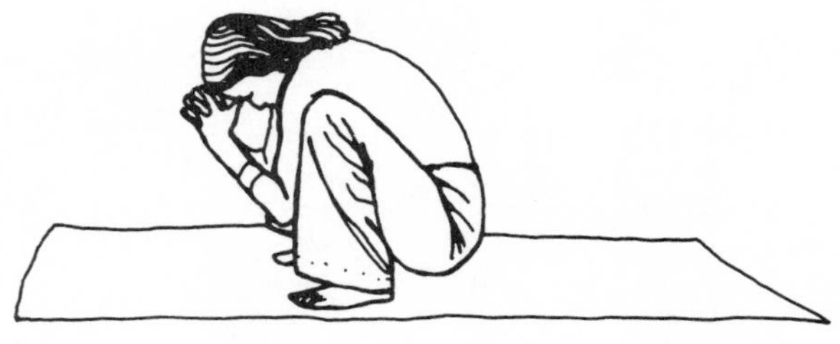

The Full Squat

Squatting is a great back release. This is really the perfect sitting posture, although in our culture it is socially unacceptable in most situations to squat. Elsewhere in the world many people do squat-sit, however, and they usually have better spines than most executives. When confined to sitting on chairs, to relieve the pressure on your lower spine from time to time, you can go in the rest room and squat, or squat by your desk if you have a private office.

In the Car

You can treat the driver to a back refresher from the backseat: do the Trapezius Squeeze on shoulder muscles by lifting and squeezing with the

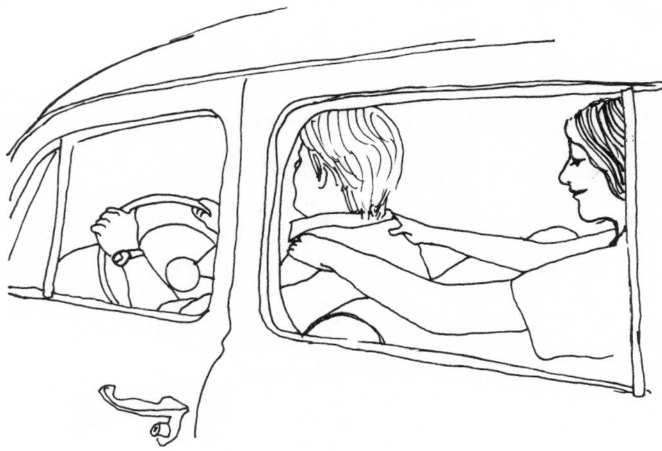

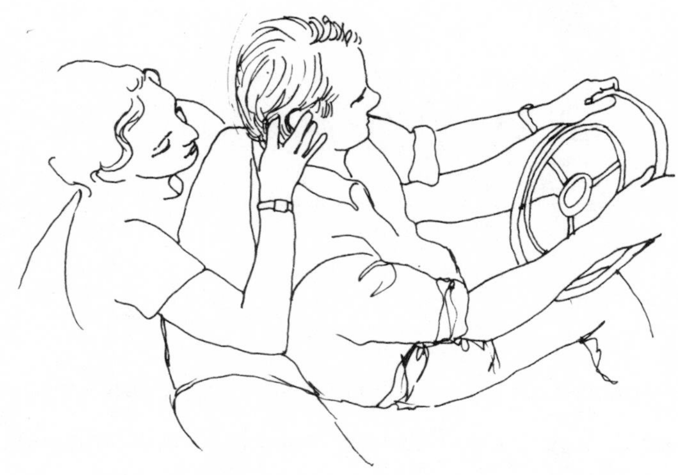

fingers and thumb of each hand. With your thumbs on the upper back muscles and your fingers above the collar bones, pinch and slide them up and off the shoulders as you squeeze. Repeat this motion rhythmically.

The neck can be released from driving tension with pressure around the base of the skull. Use your thumbs to press upward under the occipital ridge (where the skull meets the neck), bracing your elbows on the back of the front seat.

Grand Prix Exercise

Consultant to Olympic gold medal skiers and Grand Prix race drivers, Willy Dungl is a masseur and sports fitness specialist who lives in Vienna. Grand Prix drivers suffer in the extreme all the physical problems of car and plane travel: circulatory stress, static stress on spine and neck, metabolic stress from speedy travel. Here is Dungl's back muscle exercise; try it if your trip begins to feel like the Grand Prix.

Similar to a sit up, this exercise is done lying on your stomach. Lie face down over a table or bed with only legs and pelvis supported, arms clasped behind the neck, torso hanging toward the floor. Raise your torso up parallel to your hips. Then lower and repeat the lift as many times as is comfortable.

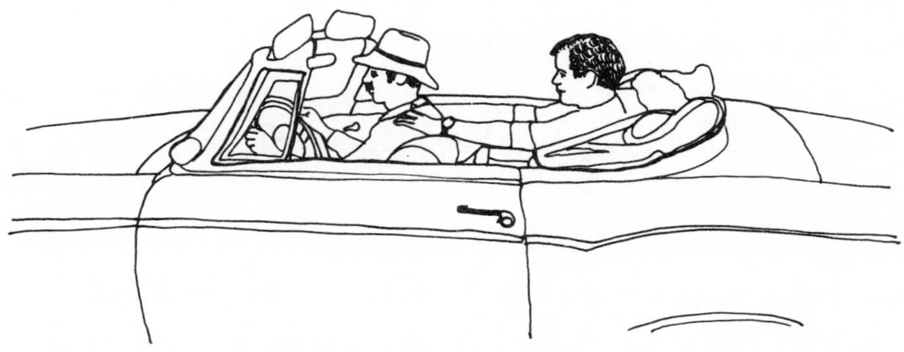

ATHLETIC BACK RUBS

Athletes continually face physical challenges that can lead to back problems. People injure themselves in amateur and professional sports activities more often and more severely than they might if they did not exercise. However, the payoffs in increased stamina, a toned physique, a more positive attitude, improved healing capacity, and better resistance to disease more than make up for the problems of exercise injury.

Suppleness Is All

Most professional athletes build preventive work into their regimes, and back rubs have become an important prelude to a top-notch athletic workout. As a group, professional athletes have a lower incidence of back problems than the rest of the population. I'm convinced this is because pros' muscles are strong and supple from regular exercise, and they learn how to move so that they do not strain their backs.

Football players and race car drivers have a higher incidence of back injuries than other athletes. Football players are frequently less supple than athletes in other fields. Race car drivers do their work sitting down, and their spines endure tremendous high-speed G-forces. Runners also often develop back problems from bad shoes, incorrect stride, and the constant pounding on the disk spaces during running.

Back pains and injuries are largely muscular. Back rubs feel good when you are recuperating from sports injuries and encourage healing. After the initial rest period, you can begin a new exercise routine that is good for your back, and back massage can play a vital role in this process.

Practice Preventive Medicine

Preventive activity should focus on improving circulation to the muscles; this delivers more oxygen, necessary for their proper functioning, and clears out the lactic acid that builds up in the muscles. Gentle muscle stimulation before the stretching phase of a workout helps prevent muscle strain, so massage is important before as well as after exercising. Stretching muscles and tendons too far—or when they are chilled—causes minute tears. These tears result in the formation of scar tissue and render the muscle less flexible.

Use the Buddy System

A warm-up buddy system is helpful. A brief exchange of back rubs before a workout warms up the tissues, improves circulation, and helps prevent injuries. The resulting relaxation also improves your performance. After an exercise period, back rubs can be incorporated into your cool-down phase. The back has some of the longest muscles in the body, and the nerves of the spine reach to all parts of the body. Thus, a back rub can improve the responses of your whole body. You may not be a pro athlete, but you can enjoy a pro warmup with a back rub!

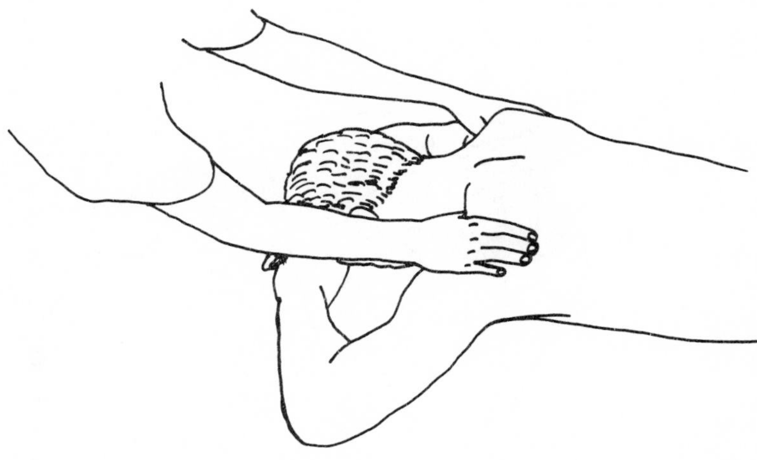

A Back Rub for Athletes

15 minutes

V Press—8 sets each side, shoulders to hips

Trapezius Press—1 set

Spine Squeeze—1

Blade Rub—1 each side

The Middle Back: The Rib Map—1

Pinching—lower back & buttocks

Pelvis Pockets—1 set

V Press—1 hips to shoulders

Spine Snake—1 down

Bear Walk—2 up & down

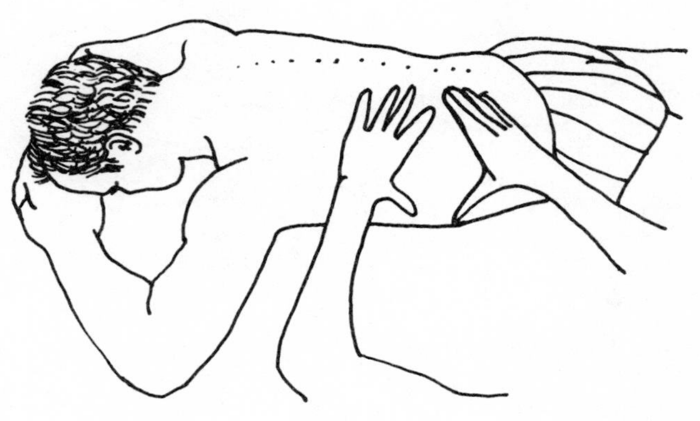

V Press

Stand at your friend's side. Spread the thumb and forefinger of one hand as far apart as possible. Run your open hand down one side of the back. Move swiftly and use only the thumb, forefinger, and the taut V of skin stretched between for hard pressure on the muscle.

As you near the hip, begin bringing your other hand, thumb and forefinger spread in the same fashion, back up the same route. Then again draw the first hand down and the second hand up and so on, developing a comfortable rhythm. Spread your feet several feet apart, so you can lean your entire body back and forth along with the movement of your hands. Stroke up and down eight times. Walk to your friend's other side and do the same. The rocking motion you achieve can make this stroke very enjoyable to give and to receive.

Trapezius Press

Stand above your friend's head. Resting your palms lightly on either shoulder, use your thumbs to apply gradual pressure along the trapezius

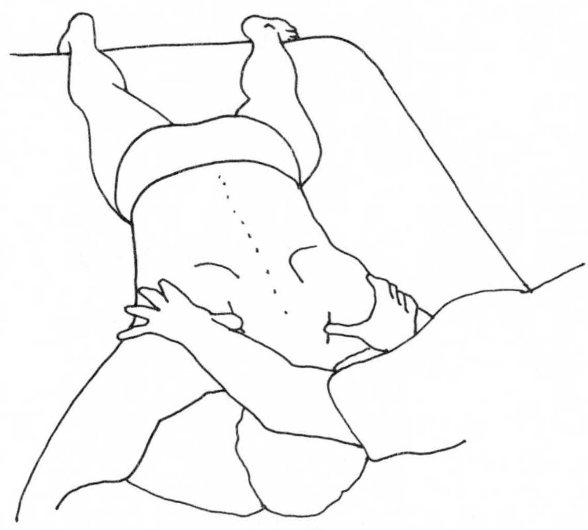

muscle running from the neck to the outer edges of the shoulders. When you find a spot on the muscle that feels tight, spend more time there to relieve the tension. Thumb pressure should be applied very gradually until you reach a level that you want to be still and hold for a while. When you release the pressure, do it as gradually as you applied it. Don't hurt your friend. Pain causes tension in the muscle. Apply pressure up to the point of soreness. Then wait for your friend's muscles to relax and soften; then move on to the next spot. You can use this pressure technique also on the muscles of the upper back between the spine and the shoulder blades.

Spine Squeeze

Place your thumbs on the muscles on either side of the spine at the base of the neck. Lean your weight firmly but gradually down onto your hands and angle your finger pressure slightly in toward the space between two vertebrae. Hold this pressure a moment. Then release gradually and move your thumbs in between the next lower vertebrae. Repeat this pressure and release between the vertebrae along the whole spinal column. Take care that you don't skip a vertebra. When you reach the waist area, just below the ribs, be sure to angle your thumbs toward each other. Do not press down on the spine at the curve of the back. On the sacrum (the arrowhead bone at the base of the spine) you can press down again. When you reach the sacrum, lean your weight into your thumbs and slide them all the way up to the neck, staying in the grooves on either side of the spine between the spine and the long muscles paralleling it.

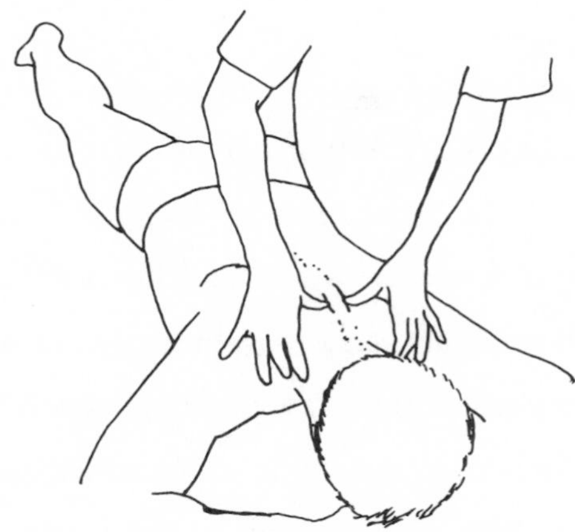

Blade Rub

To reach the muscles of the shoulder blade area well you need to raise the blade while massaging. Gently place your friend's right hand, palm up,

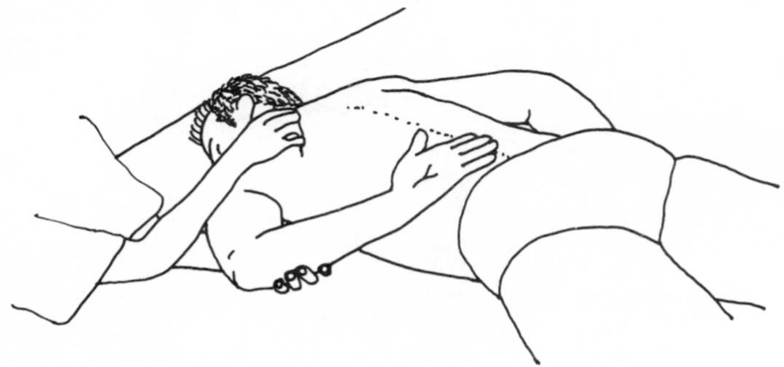

on the small of his or her back, and slide your right forearm under the shoulder until your palm cups the elbow, and the shoulder rests in the crook of your arm. Press and slide the fingertips of your left hand along the arc now opened up between the spine and the blade. Make several smooth, semicircular strokes around the edge of the blade. Then massage the same area, making small circles with your fingertips. Slide your arm gently away from your friend's arm, and lower the hand so that it lies flat on the table or bed again. Move to your friend's left side and repeat this stroke.

The Middle Back: The Rib Map

Use the tips and sides of your thumbs to define the muscles in the space between each rib. Start at the vertebrae just below the shoulder blades. Lean your weight slightly into your friend's back. Keep your thumbs on either side of the vertebrae. Slide your thumbs away from each other, defining the area between each rib across your friend's back and down his or her sides. Slide your thumbs all the way down to the table or bed. Then lift your hands and bring them back to either side of the spine. Start on the next rib and work your way down all the ribs.

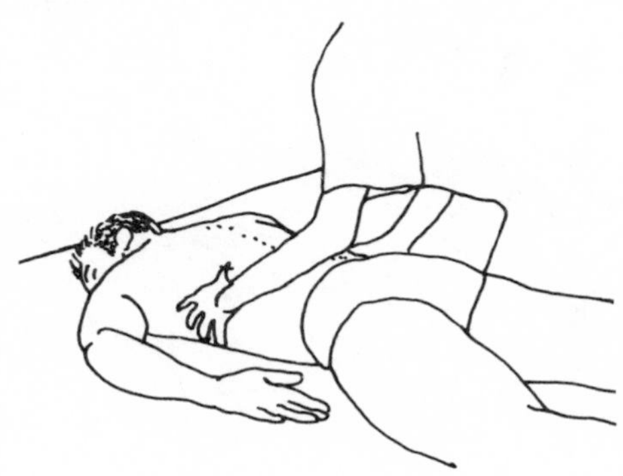

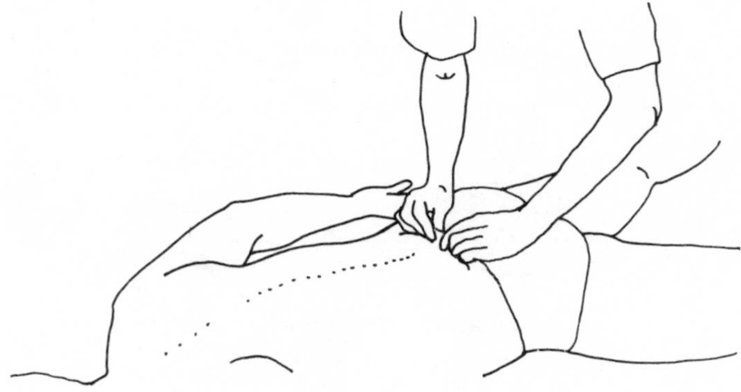

Pinching

The motion of the pinching stroke is to grip a fold of skin between the thumb and fingertips of each hand, lifting and squeezing the skin. This should be done firmly and gently with both hands. You are stimulating the tiny nerves in the skin. You can do a "pinching" massage all over the body, but there are certain areas where it feels especially good. One of these is the lower back. Sit at your friend's side, parallel to the hips and facing the head. Begin the pinching on the buttocks and continue across the sacrum and lower back. The area around the sacrum is full of nerves that spread into the pelvis, and it is often tense. Work like an inchworm, lifting folds of skin between your thumbs and fingers all around the edges of the sacrum bone, on top of it, and up around the waist.

Pelvis Pockets

Sitting beside your friend near the thighs, work on the area around each leg where the thigh moves into the pelvis. Deep massage here is very relaxing for the pelvis and the leg muscles. Use the balls of your thumbs

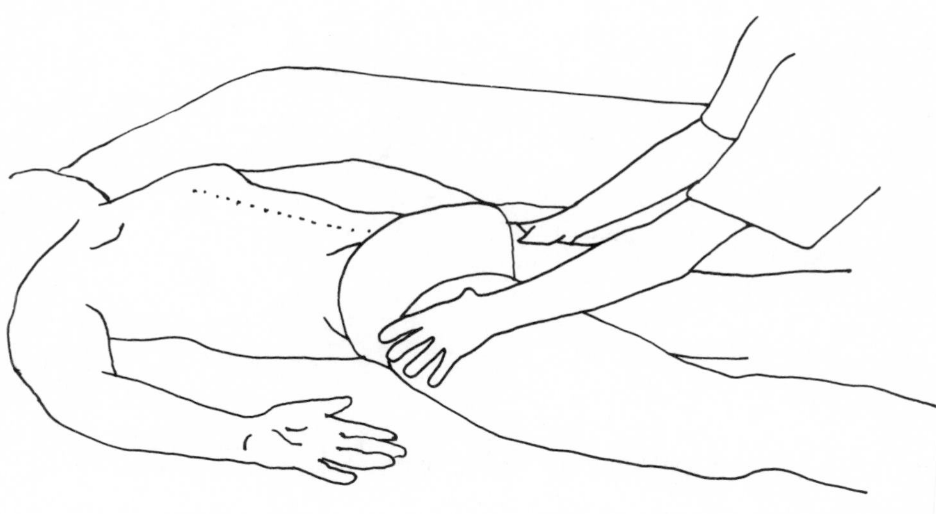

or your fingertips. You can work on one leg at a time or both legs at once. Locate small depressions at the top of the thigh around the pelvic bone or sitting bone. Press in with your fingertips toward the pelvic bone. When you are in as far as you can go, rotate your fingers in small circles on the spot. Work systematically from the crease of the inner thigh up across the back of the leg and onto the side of the hip.

V Press

Repeat the V Press stroke you started with, this time moving from the hips to the shoulders.

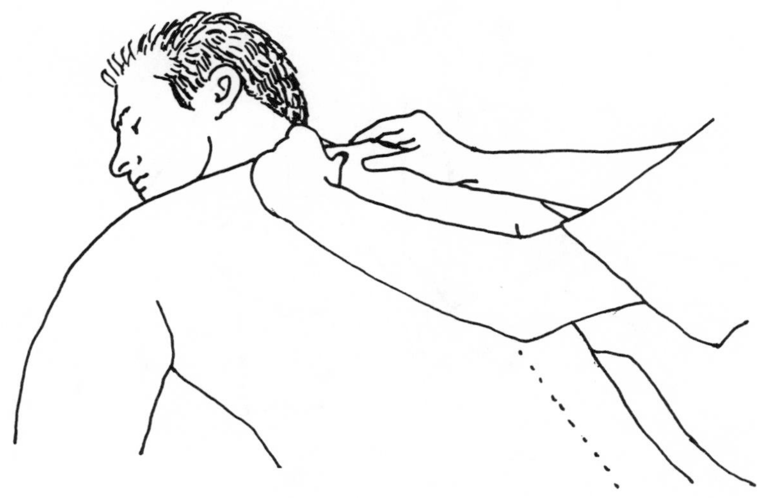

Spine Snake

Begin this movement at the top of the back by squeezing and lifting the skin over the spine with your thumbs and forefingers. Begin a rolling motion, by sliding your thumbs up toward your knuckles, that you will continue all the way to the tailbone. By this point in the massage, some of the oil on the back has been absorbed. That's good, because the Spine Snake is easier to do when the back's not too slippery. Gently grasp a roll of skin and then roll it along all the way up. On the receiving end, this is very releasing because it feels as though you are lifting nerves that may be tense and relieving pressure from the spine. Do this roll once down the spine. Try to make the stroke continuous. If you lift the next area of skin before completely letting go of the first, you can make it feel as though you are making one long roll along the whole spine. Mmmmm.

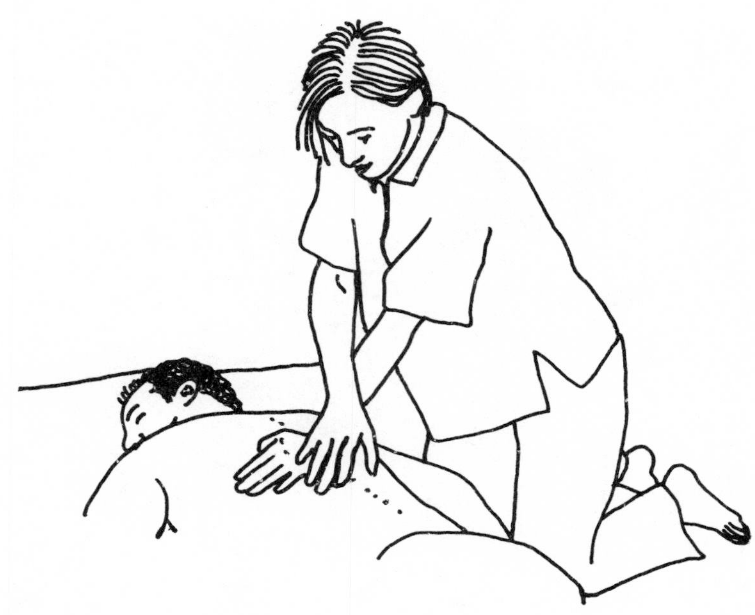

Bear Walk

Reach across and lean and press one palm against the top of the farther side of your friend's back, the heel of your hand just to the far side of the spine. Next place your other hand beside the first and below it and press. Keep crossing your hands over and pressing on the muscle as though walking down the back. Move down one side of the back over the buttock and, having crossed over to your friend's other side, up the opposite side of the back. Repeat several times.

Slow your rhythm gradually as you approach the end of the stroke. Finish the massage at the top of the back with several strokes across the trapezius muscles, sweeping your palms lightly from either side of the neck out toward the shoulders.

PREGNANCY BACK RUBS

If you want to give a pregnant friend a special baby shower treat, offer her a back rub. During pregnancy the weight of the baby puts extra strain on a woman's back muscles. A back rub can be especially soothing.

Belly muscles are major spine supporters. They wrap around your waist area and attach to the spine along the ribs and lower back. The majority of backaches are partially caused by weak or strained belly muscles. This is why pregnant women are often plagued with backaches.

A back rub is the most sensible massage to give your pregnant friend because you don't want to press on her belly. You also should use relatively light pressure on her back, except on small, finger-sized areas when you are applying shiatsu pressure. The back rub should be done with the woman lying on her side. Placing pillows between her knees and at her neck will make her more comfortable.

The following back rub will relax the muscles most stressed during pregnancy and improve circulation to strained muscles that are under pressure and ache because of decreased oxygen supply.

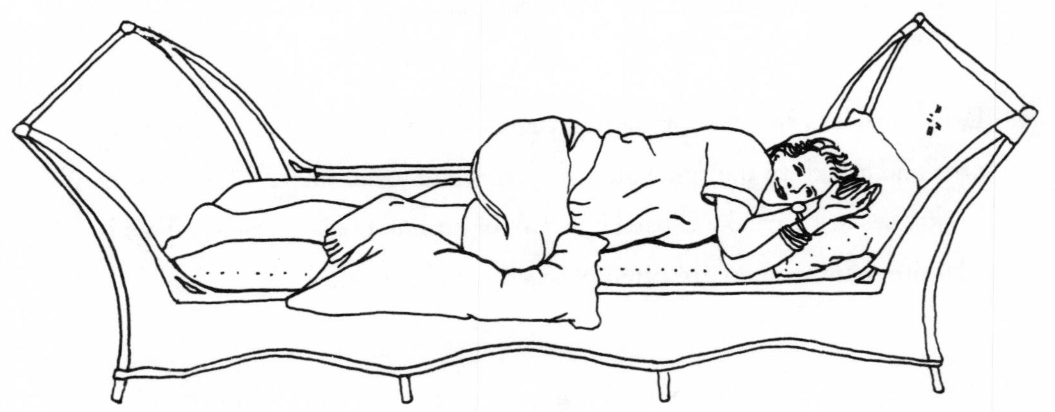

A Pregnancy Back Rub

15 minutes

Thumb Slide — 1 set
Spine Lift — 1 down spine
Blade Lift — 1 set
Sacrum Pressure Points — 1 set
Vertebrae Circles — 1 up spine
Spine Sweep — 6

A PREGNANCY BACK RUB

These strokes can be performed with oil, or without if your friend is clothed. She should be lying on her side.

Thumb Slide

Using both thumbs, make a firm, overlapping motion on the muscles of the upper back. Move from the area between the shoulder blades up onto the neck. Press one thumb down just before lifting the other, as though you were twiddling your thumbs on the muscle while moving across it. Work on one side of the spine at a time. You can end this stroke with several sweeps of your thumbs from either side of the spine outward toward the shoulder blades.

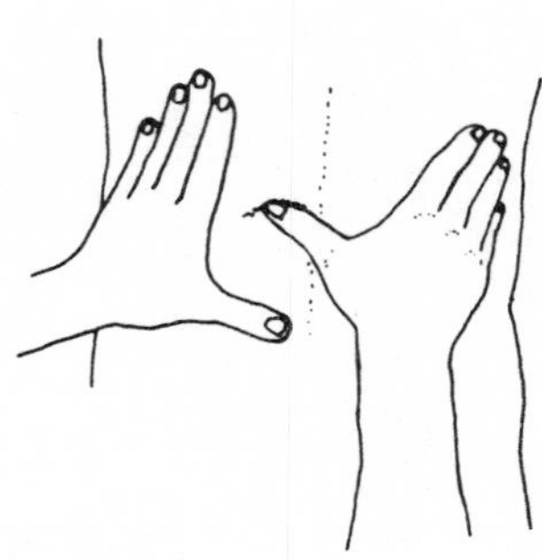

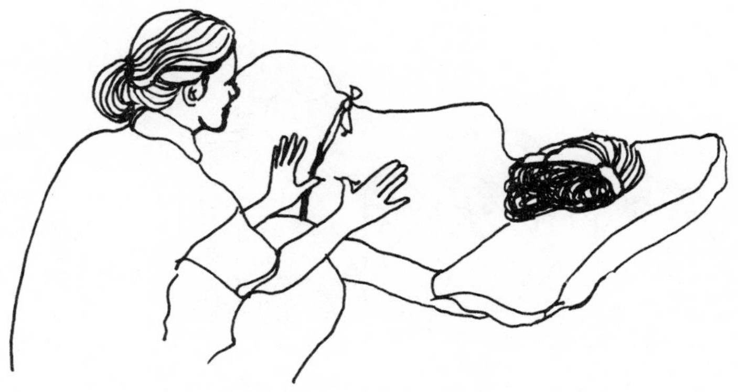

Spine Lift

This stroke moves from the upper back down to the sacrum (the arrowhead bone at the base of the spine) and should be synchronized with your friend's natural breathing. Press and lift as she exhales; release as she inhales. Place both your thumbs parallel to and under the vertebrae several inches apart. Wait for your friend's next exhalation to begin and then lean forward into your hands and angle your weight up so that your friend's spine lifts slightly away from the bed. After three or four breaths, lean back as she inhales and release your pressure, allowing the spine to come down again. Then slide your hands an inch or so lower. Repeat this lifting and release all the way down the spine. This stroke often allows compressed vertebrae to spread out and relax into place.

Blade Lift

Have your friend position her head slightly forward with the chin tucked under, her arms relaxed across her chest. The leg lying on the bed should

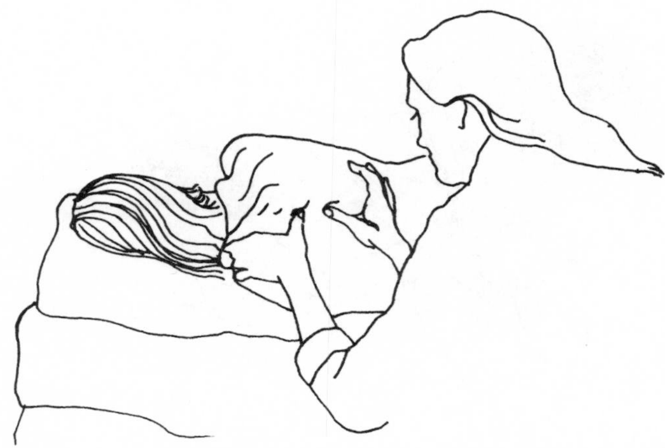

be fairly straight, while the upper leg should be bent at the knee to support her. In this position the shoulder and shoulder blade are pulled by gravity toward the bed. Place your fingertips or your thumbs under the shoulder blade. If your friend's muscles are relaxed enough, position your fingertips in between the shoulder blade and the back. The muscles that hold the trapezius to the back often get tense. Massage these muscles in a slow half circle from the top of the shoulder along the shoulder blade toward the ribs. If she wants, your friend can roll over, so you can repeat the same stroke on the other side.

Sacrum Pressure Points

Shiatsu is a form of Japanese pressure point massage based on the same energy system as acupuncture. Although the complete system requires training, you can use a simple version of pressure point massage for relaxing effects.

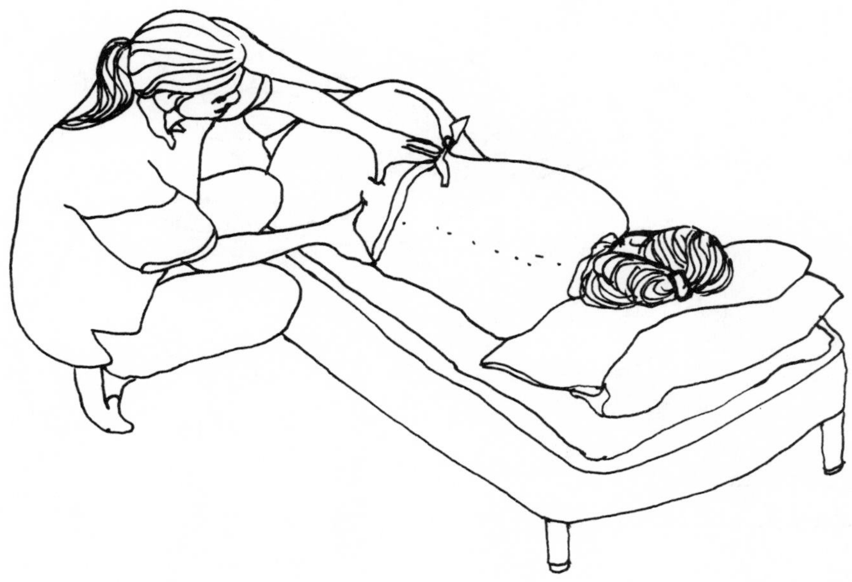

Stand beside your friend's hips. Lean your weight into your arms as you press your thumbs on either side of one of your friend's sacral vertebrae. Gradually angle more of your weight into your hands.

Release the pressure just as gradually as you applied it, so that your hands come out of your friend's muscles very slowly. Then move your thumbs down to the next sacral vertebra. Apply the pressure of your body weight again. Work your way from the top of the sacrum to the tip. Then apply the same type of gradual pressure to the outsides of the sacrum, from your friend's waist down to the tailbone. The pressure should be deep but not painful. If it is painful you are pressing either too quickly or too hard for her muscles to relax with the pressure. You might not be in quite the right spot, so shift your position and try another spot.

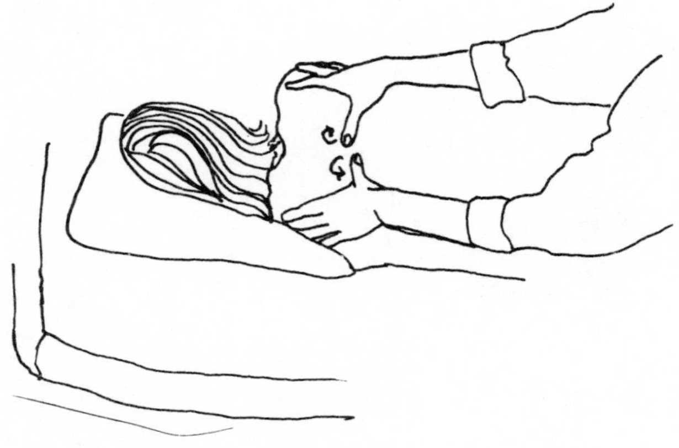

Vertebrae Circles

Use the tips and sides of your thumbs to define the muscles in the space between each pair of vertebrae. Start at the sacral vertebrae in the lower back. Lean your weight slightly into your friend's back. Keep your thumbs on either side of the vertebra. Slide your thumbs in small circles, defining the area between each pair of vertebrae all the way up your friend's back.

Spine Sweep

This is a simple stroke that usually feels wonderful. It also has a way of connecting all the separate strokes you've done with one sweep, so it makes a pleasant ending stroke. Place your palms on your friend's shoulders. Draw them along the muscles on either side of the spine down the back and over the hips. As you cross the hips, angle your hands away from

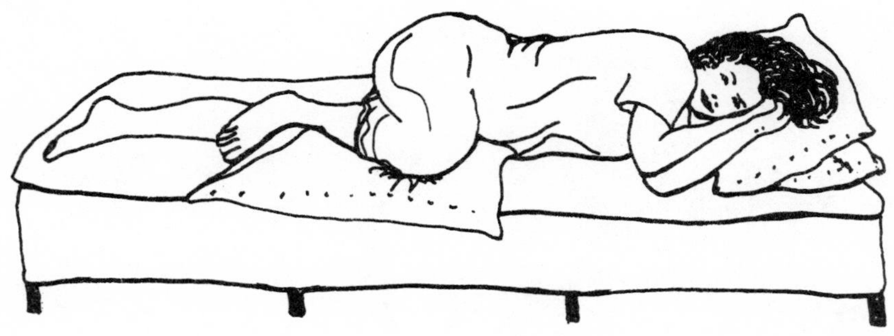

each other and lift them off her body. Return your palms to the shoulders and repeat the sweep with light, swift strokes.

A BACK RUB FOR BABY

Infants love to be massaged as much as anyone else. However, they may show their enthusiasm by moving around a lot, so you'll have to become adept at giving back rubs to a moving object. Soothing touch helps stimulate nerve and muscle development and improves coordination in infants.

Infants are in a heightened state of sensory awareness compared with adults, and sensitive massage following the shape of the body helps an infant increase the sense of self and define the boundaries between self and the rest of the world. Babies who lack touching can become depressed or ill, and develop more slowly.

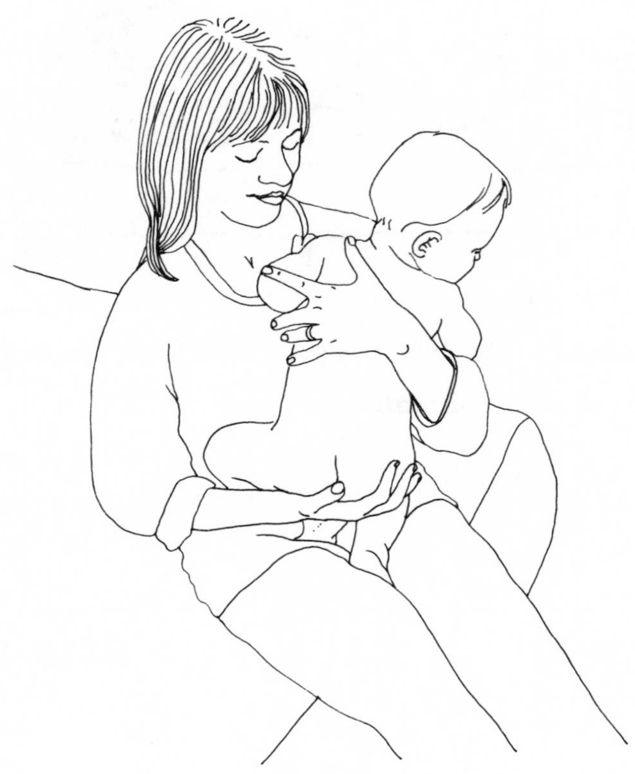

Back rubs are reassuring to an upset child, to calm them after an accident, to help put them to sleep, or simply to reaffirm the bond between parent and child. A back rub for a baby should be relaxed, gentle, and in the spirit of yet another form of play you can share with each other.

The infant massage techniques described here are aimed at encouraging the baby's sense of physical strength and joy, stimulating sensory and motor development, and increasing the positive bonding between parent and child.

In Chinese acupuncture, health is assured by the balance of yin and yang elements in the body. Yin is the system of the receptive aspects of the body, symbolized by the moon. Yang is the system of active elements in the body, symbolized by the sun.

The back of the body, the outsides of the legs, and the backs of the arms are considered yang. To follow the principles of acupuncture, you move your strokes down yang meridians and up yin meridians. This means you should move strokes along the backs of arms from wrists to the shoulders. Move strokes on baby's back from shoulders to hips.

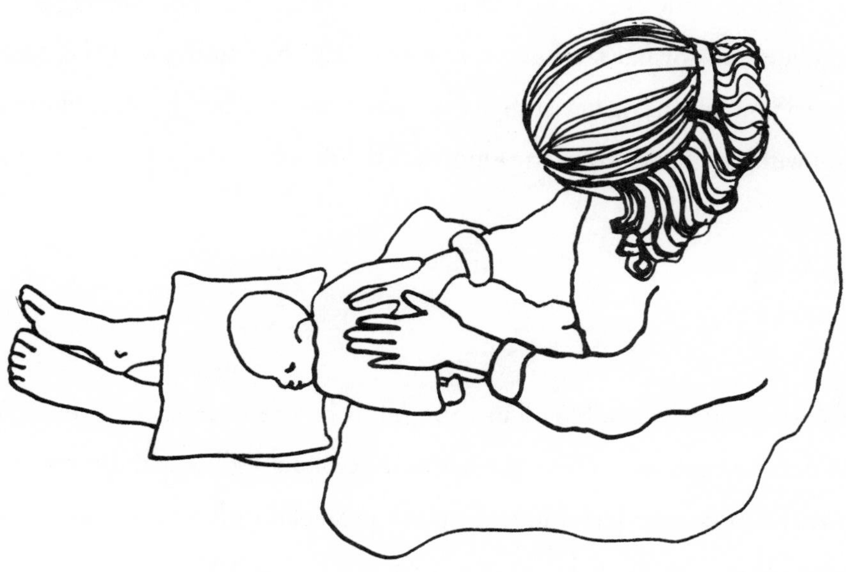

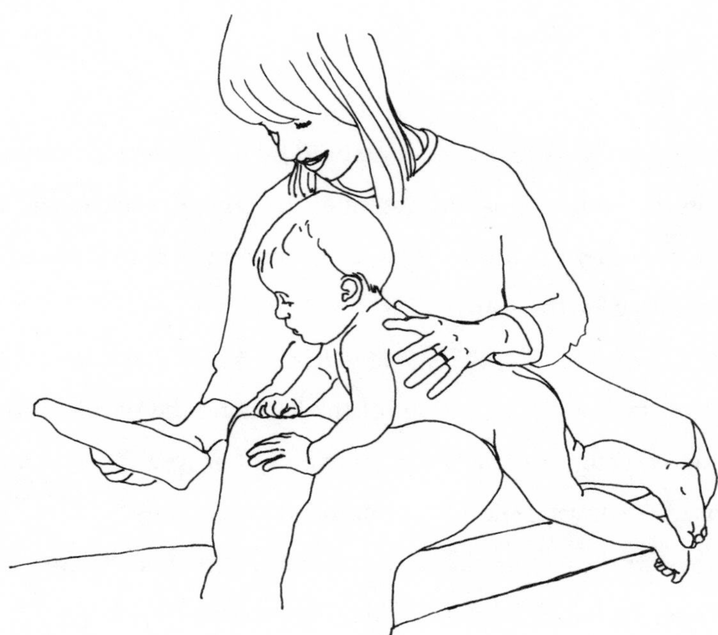

Positions

Massage the baby in any natural position that's comfortable: holding the baby against your chest while sitting and stroking the back; having the baby lie on his or her stomach across your lap; having the baby lie, feet toward you, on his or her stomach on your outstretched legs. Support the baby with one hand while stroking with the other.

Lubricants

Warm a pure vegetable oil in your palms before massaging. French clay powder also makes a pleasant lubricant. Stroking lightly without oil or powder can be wonderful too. Or you can stroke with a pure cotton pad. Some babies like the tickle of a very soft baby brush.

Stroke with your fingertips down the baby's backbone from neck to buttocks. This is a soothing way to start. The following strokes can be done in any sequence.

Stroke from the top of the head down the neck and right side of the back. Then continue stroking down the back outer side of the right leg to the foot.

Move to the back of the right wrist, and glide up the arm to the right shoulder and the top of the head.

Stroke from the head to the neck and down the complete body length, over the left side of the baby's back and over the left outer side of the left leg to the foot.

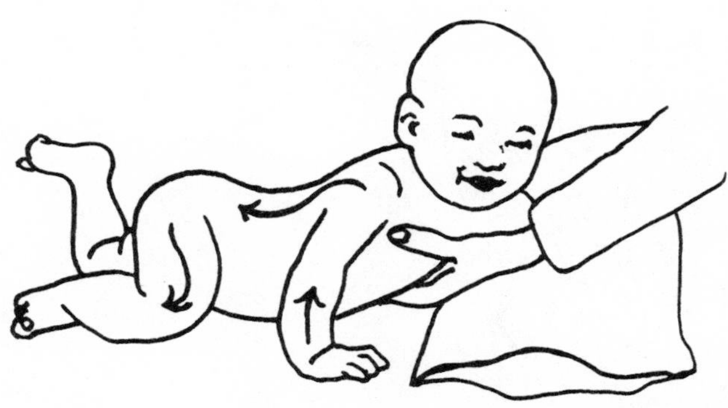

Then glide from the back of the left wrist up the arm to the left shoulder and rest your palm in the center of the back between the baby's shoulder blades.

Make light, rhythmic circles on the upper back, occasionally stroking down the entire length of the spine to the baby's tailbone.

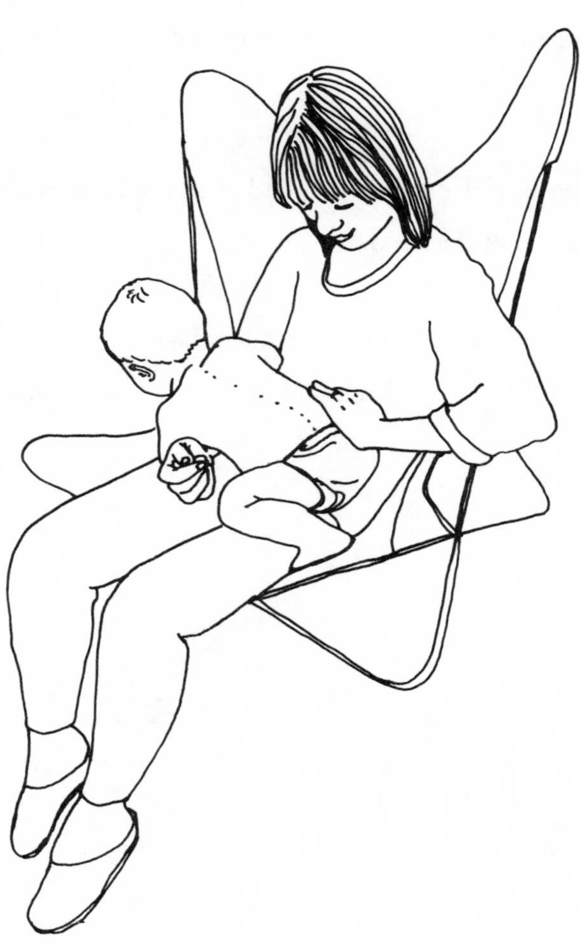

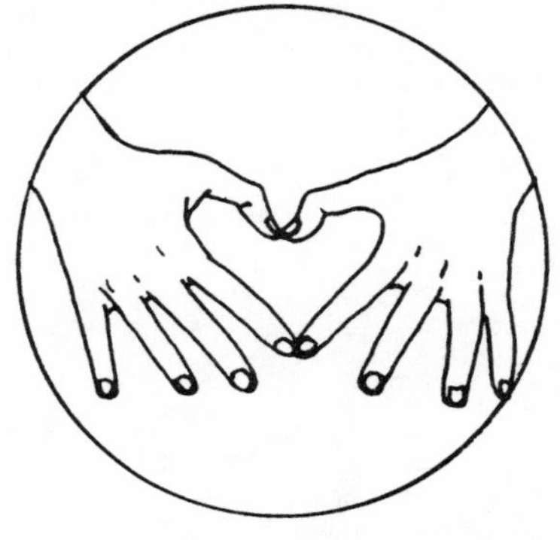

SPECIAL OCCASIONS

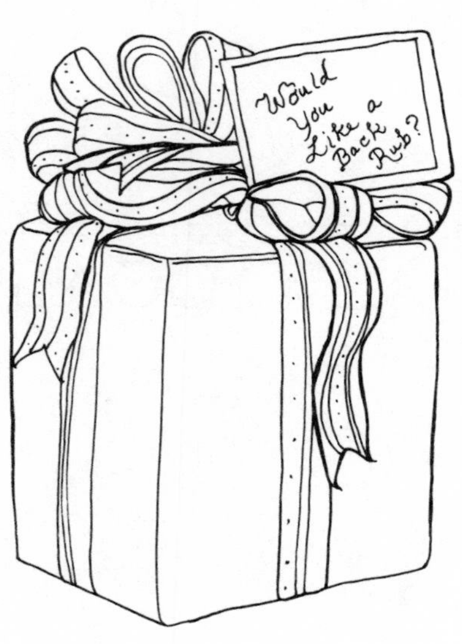
Would
You
Like a
Back
Rub?

OILS, HERBS & EXOTICS

Make any day a special occasion by giving a special treat. Along with a back rub, oils, herbs, and powders in pretty bottles and boxes make lovely, luxurious gifts, for others and for yourself.

Oils

You can mix excellent massage oil yourself. Combine one part almond oil and four parts unprocessed vegetable oil (from health food or grocery stores) with several drops of scent oil.

1. **Obtain especially fine back rub oils**

   Almond

   Avocado

   Lanolin

   Safflower

   Sunflower

2. **Add fragrance oil**

   Almond

   Chocolate

Cinnamon
Lavender
Mint
Musk
Peach
Rose
Sandalwood

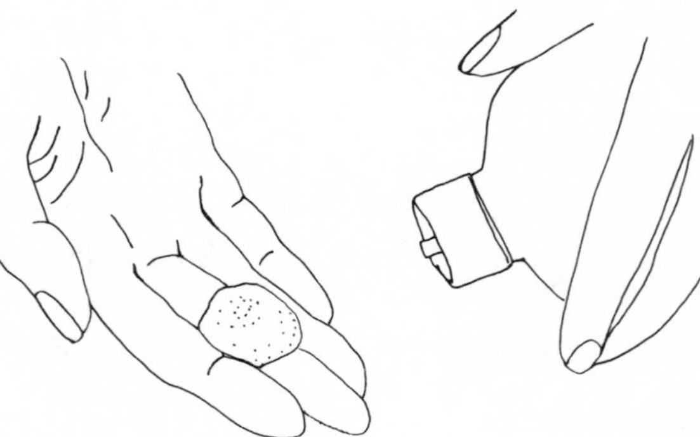

Remember to keep the scent minimal. When you pour the oil out and cover your friend, the scent will smell stronger than it does confined in the bottle.

3. **Add skin treats**

   A teaspoon (or more if you like) of these special oils will enhance the health and beauty effects of the vegetable oils:

   Wheat germ oil for vitamin E and for removing skin discolorations
   Aloe vera oil for smoothing and healing the skin
   Lanolin oil for moisturizing
   Primrose oil for toning and adding vitamins
   Jojoba oil for moisturizing
   Apricot kernel oil for moisturizing
   Na-PCA for clearing up wrinkles
   Honey for tightening the pores

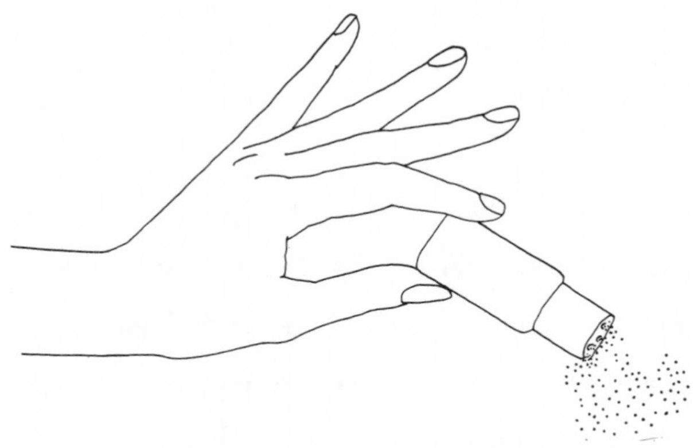

Powders

Most soothing of all powders to the skin is French clay powder, white or green. French clay powder is nonallergenic, absorbs odors, and detoxifies acids and irritants in the skin. French clay powders come unscented or in lovely blends, such as rose or mixed flowers.

PREMASSAGE BODY RUBS

Premassage body rubs prepare the skin for receiving beneficial massage oils and relax tense muscles. Try almond meal or cornmeal rubs to cleanse pores. Rinse off in a warm shower to open pores to oils and herbs.

Milk and Meal

In a steamy sauna, apply a mixture of buttermilk and sea salt to a hot washcloth, and scrub your back. The salt cleans the pores and the milk supplies ingredients beneficial to your skin. Yogurt and almond meal mixed make a slightly less abrasive cleanser. Be sure to include your upper arms and the back of your neck in your scrub. Rinse with cool water to close your pores again.

Milk and Honey

The ancient panacea of milk and honey is still an unbeatable treat. You can apply milk, yogurt or honey directly to your skin. First the milk moistens the skin. Then apply honey to tighten it. Leave each on awhile so it can be absorbed. Rinse off with warm water.

A Delicious Astringent

Take two egg whites whisked with several drops of lemon juice and apply to skin. Leave for ten minutes. Rinse with warm water.

The Tingle Cure for Backaches

Try Tiger Balm, a tingling, aromatic Chinese ointment that comes in beautiful jars. Apply sparingly to tense muscles. They will tingle and warm. An ancient antidote for lack of energy is to scratch Tiger Balm into your skin along your ribs and back with a piece of jade.

Anti-Backache Shower

Jeanne Rose devised an herbal treatment for low backache. Mix together handfuls of these dried herbs in a muslin bag: rosemary leaves, sage leaves, strawberry leaves, comfrey root, comfrey leaves, lavender buds. Close the bag and soak it thoroughly in water. In a hot shower, rub the herb-filled sack on your skin from your feet to your lower back with a circular motion. As you rub, alternate the water temperature on your lower back from one minute of hot spray to half a minute of cold spray. End the shower with a quick cold rinse.

Sun Rub

Place a cube of solid scented oil, such as coconut or cocoa butter, in the middle of your friend's back while he or she is lying in the sun. Allow the sun to melt the cube. Then give your friend a back rub.

Backlights

For daring social moments, try commercial skin creams that sparkle. Halston makes a lovely skin sparkle, as do many other companies. Spread it on your back and dazzle them coming and going!

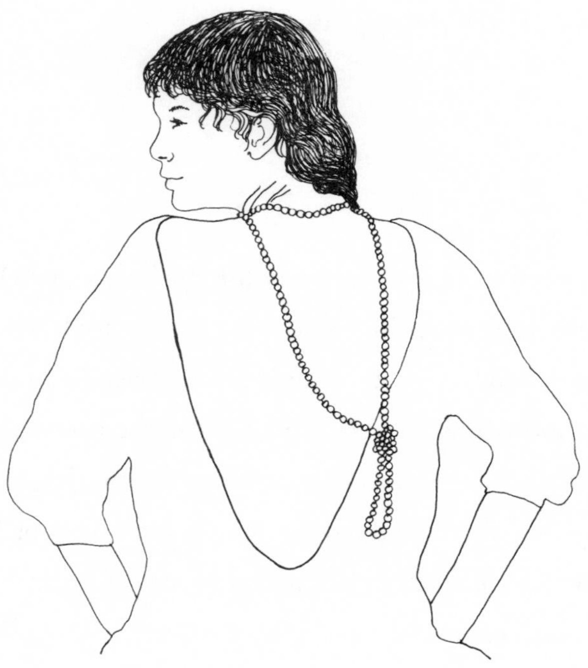

HOLIDAY BACK RUBS

The best gift is not necessarily the most expensive; it is the one that makes the person feel best. The most successful gift makes the receiver feel appreciated and affirmed in a personal way. A back rub is a gift that is available to any budget, and it can impart a sense of great luxury.

Promise Anything, but Give a Back Rub

Consider giving your friend a Back Rub IOU. You can make a special card and put it in an envelope to mail or place it in a gift box and wrap.

On an old-fashioned holiday, give an old-fashioned gift. On many major holidays, just when people are supposed to be relaxing and feeling carefree, they find themselves at their most tense and pressured. A holiday back rub helps to revive and relax your friends or relatives if they are stressed. Teach your children to give good back rubs. Giving back rubs can help a child feel effective at assisting with family responsibilities. One clever mother trained her children to work as a team; one massages her feet while the other works on her back.

Offer a back rub for parents or grandparents so some of the nurturing they gave you comes back to them.

For an outdoor treat, take a friend on a picnic and give him or her a back rub in a sunny, peaceful field. It will be a memorable holiday outing.

Don't forget your pets. Back rubs make great presents for them too!

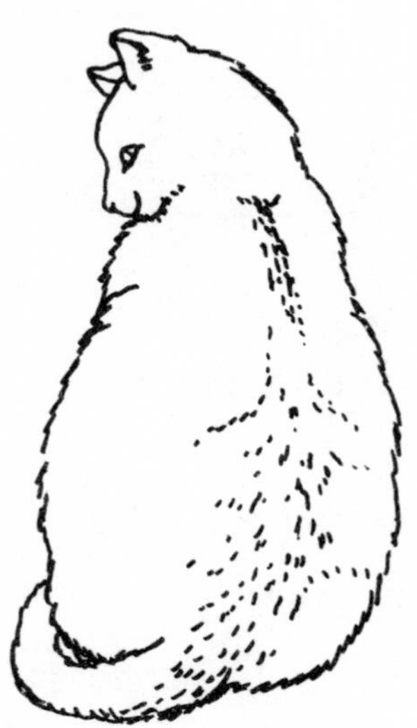

A Holiday Back Rub

15 minutes

Patting

Palm Slide — 3 sets

Trapezius Squeeze — 8

Thumbs Along the Spine — 1 set

Elbow in the Sacrum — 1 set

Bear Walk — 1 set

Spine Sweep — 8

A HOLIDAY BACK RUB

This massage is a pleasant antidote to holiday tensions. It can be done well with oils or through clothes for modest or busy friends and relatives. I've designed this back rub so the strokes are easy and fun for children to give.

Patting

Sit to one side of your friend. Using your palms and alternating hands, simply pat your friend on the back. The secret to making this a very enjoyable stroke to receive is to set up a continuous rhythm, to keep the pressure relatively light, but to use your whole palm. The pats should make a muffled clap sound. Work carefully from your friend's far shoulder down to the hips, then up the near side to the near shoulder. Continue without a break down the far side again so the patting is performed in a circular route. End on the shoulders.

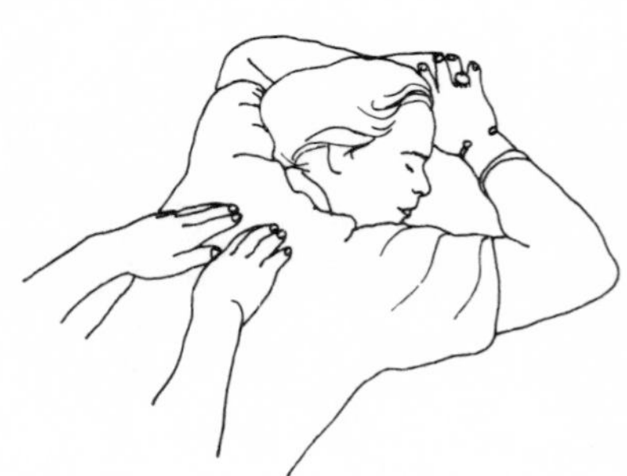

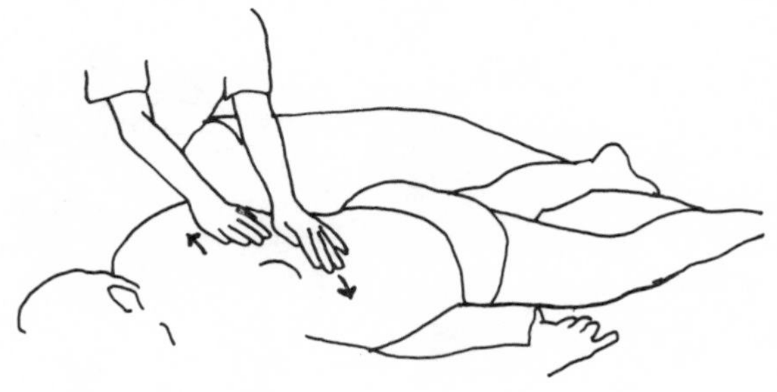

Palm Slide

Leaning onto your friend's back from beside him or her, begin slow, alternating slides with your palms across the back. Your fingertips are pointing away from you. Drag one hand toward you as the other moves away, then reverse. Work from the shoulders down the back and up again several times.

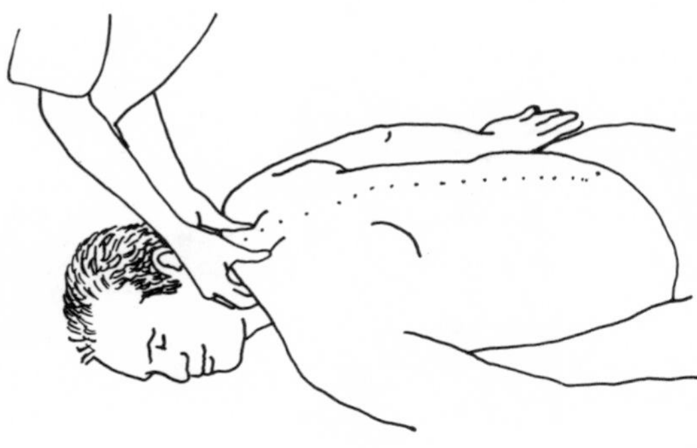

Trapezius Squeeze

On the upper back, knead the muscles curving from your friend's neck onto his or her shoulders. Working the muscles between the thumb and fingers of each hand, do both sides at once. Start with light, slow squeezes and gradually speed up and squeeze harder.

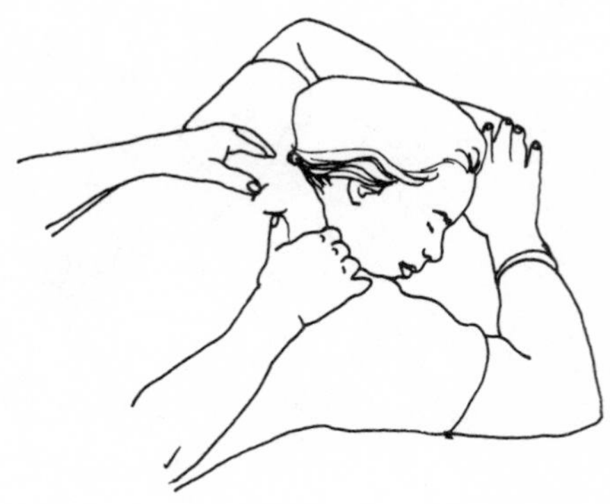

Thumbs Along the Spine

Starting between the shoulder blades, massage the long muscles to either side of the spine. Use small circular motions of your thumbs. Work down to the lower back, up, and down again. Use deep or light pressure, as your friend prefers. End at the lower back.

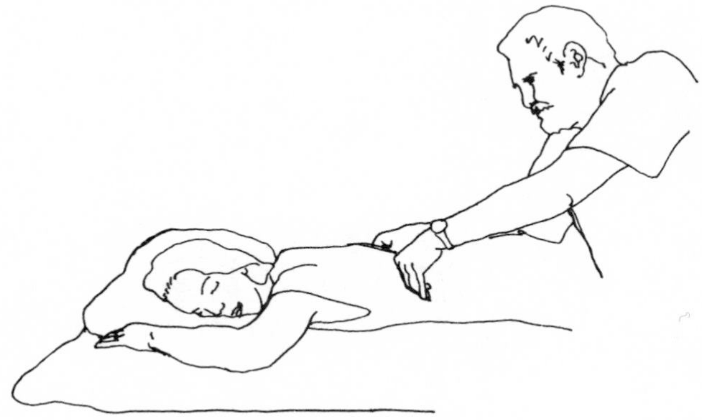

Elbow in the Sacrum

This stroke is easy to do even when you are tired from holiday activity. Place the elbow of your arm nearest your friend on top of the sacrum, the triangular, flat bone at the base of the spine. Sit your chin in your palm and rest your torso weight there so your elbow presses farther into the sacrum.

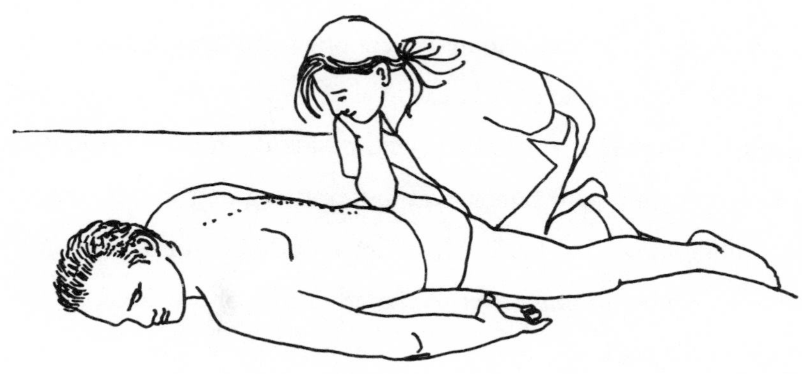

Apply pressure very gradually. Release it gradually also. Then move your elbow lower on the sacrum and repeat the pressure and release. The lower back is quite sensitive, so you may have to move to different places to find a comfortable one. Your friend will know when you reach the right spot. When done well this stroke is extremely pleasant and relaxing.

Bear Walk

It is fun for children to know the origin of this stroke's name. In some rural villages of Eastern Europe you can lie on the ground and hire a trained bear to walk on your back.

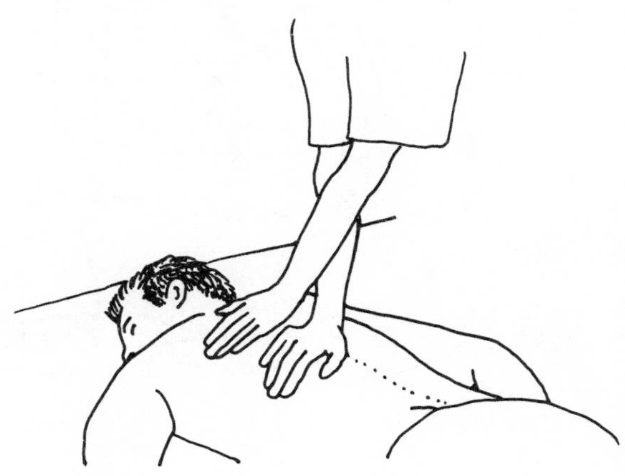

Reach across the table and lean and press one palm against the top of the farther side of your friend's back, the heel of your hand just to the far side of the spine. Next place your other hand beside the first and below it and press. Keep crossing your hands over and pressing on the muscle as though walking down the back. Move down one side of the back over the buttock and, having crossed over to the other side of the table, up the other side of the back.

Spine Sweep

Use this last stroke to connect all the others and give your friend a sense of wholeness. Place your palms on your friend's shoulders. Draw them along the muscles on either side of the spine down the back and over the hips. As you cross the hips, angle your hands away from each other and lift them off the body. Make this a continuous, sweeping motion. Return your palms to the shoulders and begin the sweep again with light, swift strokes.

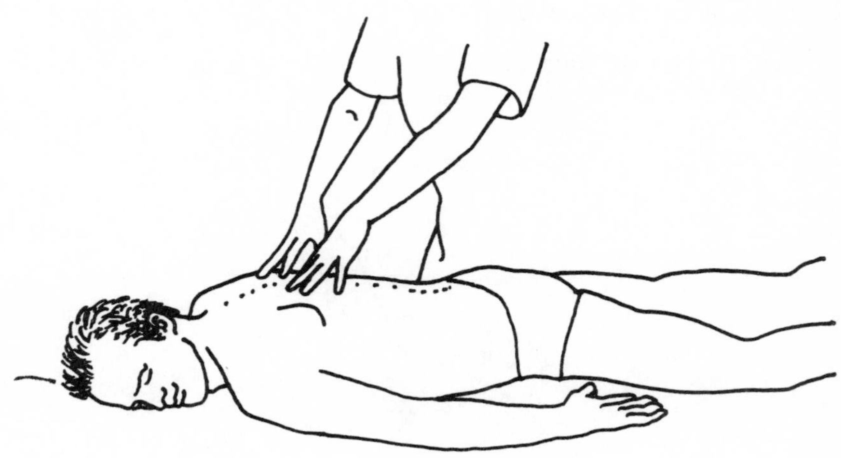

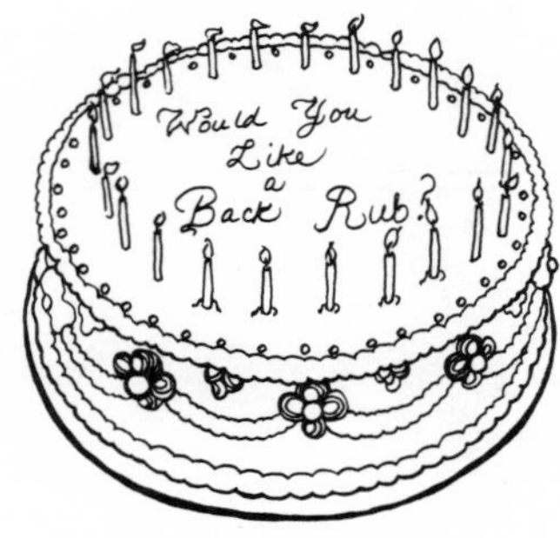

A Birthday Back Rub

1/2 hour

Main Stroke — 4

Trapezius Thumb Slide — 2 sets

Braiding — 2 down & up

Overlapping Side Palms — 1 set

Rocking Horse — 4

Big X — 4 along spine; 4 diagonally

Main Stroke — 4 waist to shoulder; last includes arms

Palm on Palm

A Birthday Back Rub

Celebrate in your birthday suit. Here's a birthday massage to give or to get that will make the receiver glad they were born.

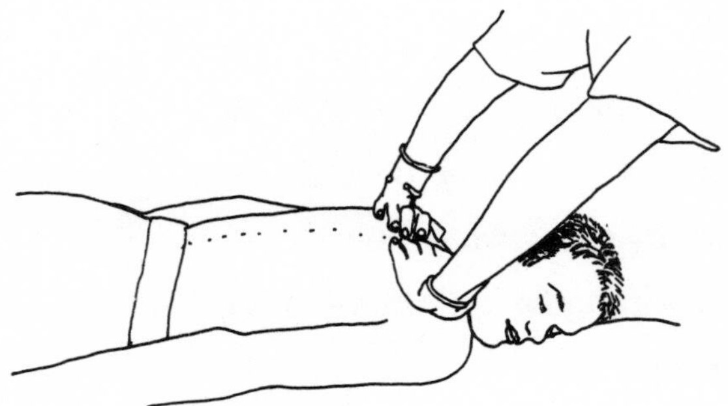

The Main Stroke

Spread some lightly scented massage oil on your friend's back, shoulders, and sides of torso.

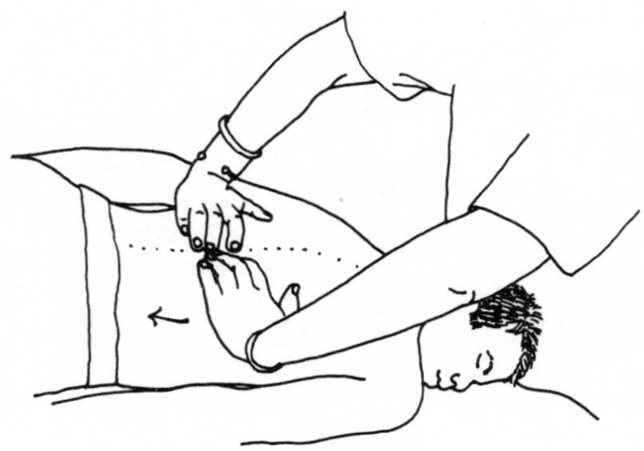

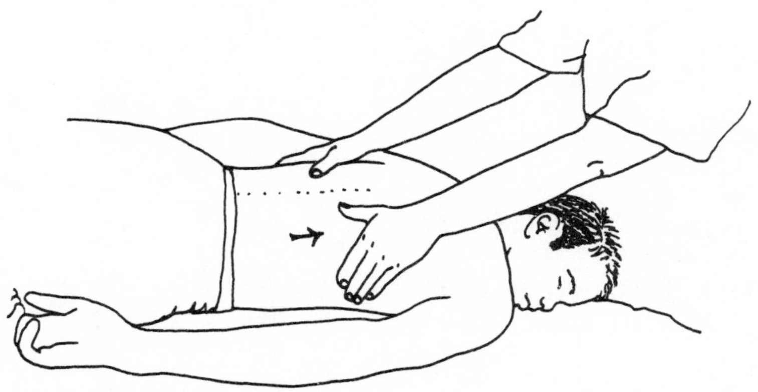

This stroke covers the whole back thoroughly. Stand above your friend's head and work from the shoulders to the waist and back up again. Place your palms on either side of the top of the back, heels of the hands on the shoulders, fingers pointing toward the spine but not on it. Slide your hands down the whole back. Maintain firm pressure, leaning forward onto your arms, pressing extra hard with your fingertips. Let your fingertips press into the furrow to either side of the spine as they move.

When you near the end of the spine, separate your hands, moving them down the sides of the hips to the table or bed. Next pull both hands along the sides of the torso up toward the shoulders almost hard enough to move your friend toward you. Before reaching the armpits, glide your hands onto the shoulders. Then pivot your fingers toward the spine to repeat the stroke.

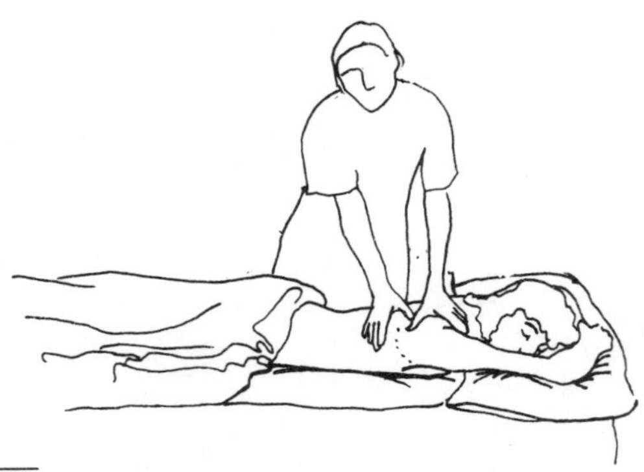

Trapezius Thumb Slide

Using both thumbs on one side of the spine, make firm, overlapping strokes. Start near the spine and work outward and downward over the muscles. Press as hard as your friend likes. You can begin this stroke on the neck and continue down the back and around the curve of a shoulder blade. Then pick your hands up, place them on the neck again, and repeat this pattern down the other side of the spine and around the other shoulder blade. Keep the thumb motion continuous and this stroke takes on a particularly relaxing roll.

Braiding

Place your right hand on your friend's right shoulder and your left hand on his left shoulder. The fingers of both your hands should point toward the table or bed. Slowly pull and press both hands, heels first, toward the spine. When the hands are about to meet, swing each hand around so that the fingers point toward each other. Moving at the same pace, press your left hand to your friend's right side and your right hand to the left side. Your forearms will form an X as your hands pass over the spine. Your fin-

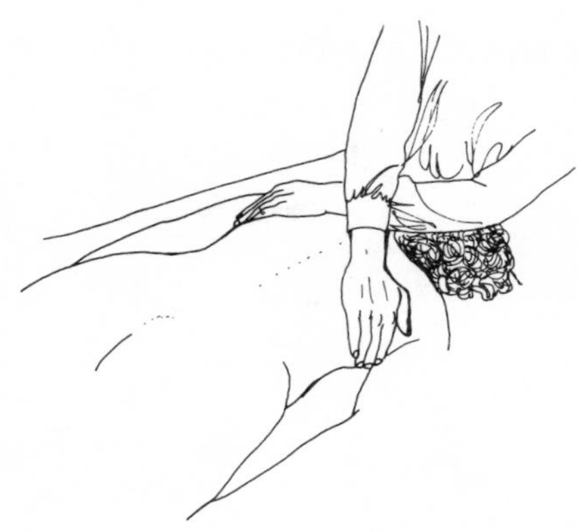

gertips will reach the table or bed. Drawing your hands a little farther down the back, begin the crossing sequence again. Make your way down and up the back in a smooth, continuous motion. Start with a very slow rhythm and gradually speed up.

Overlapping Side Palms

Move to your friend's side for this stroke and stand at his or her waist. Reach across and place your palms on the side opposite you. Pull first one hand, then the other, up from the table or bed, fingers pointing downward, in a slow, hand-over-hand rhythm. Each pull begins just as the other is

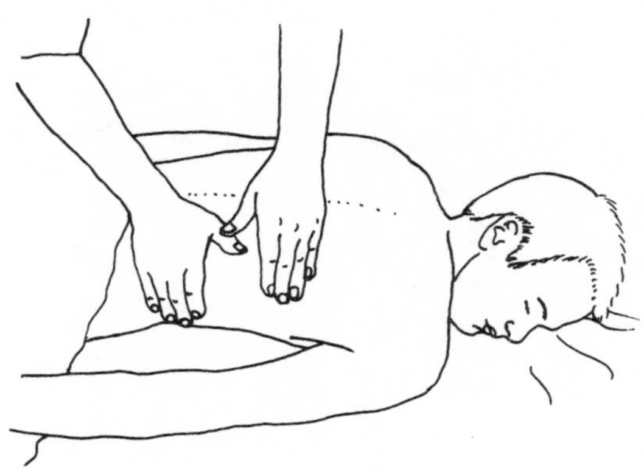

about to finish. Starting on the hip, work up to the armpit and then back again. Then move around the table or bed to begin the stroke on the opposite side.

Rocking Horse

This is one of the rare strokes that moves along the spine itself. Stand or sit to your friend's right side at the waist. Place your right palm on the sacrum, fingers pointing toward the head. Cross and cover this hand with your left palm, fingers pointing toward you. Glide your two hands as a unit up the spine, keeping a steady, moderate pressure. (Never press hard directly on the spine.) At the top of the spine, reverse the motion and draw your hands to the waist again, this time digging the tips of your forefinger and middle finger into the grooves on either side of the spine. As you slide down, you can press a lot harder than on the way up. When you reach the sacrum, move up the spine again with your flat palm. This stroke's name comes from the rocking motion you achieve if the up and down strokes are done continuously.

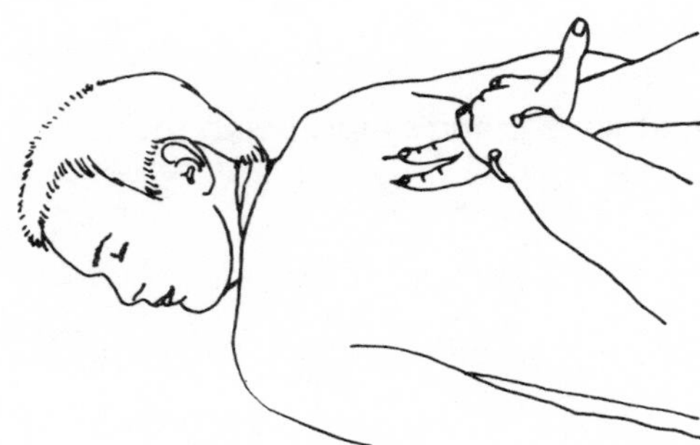

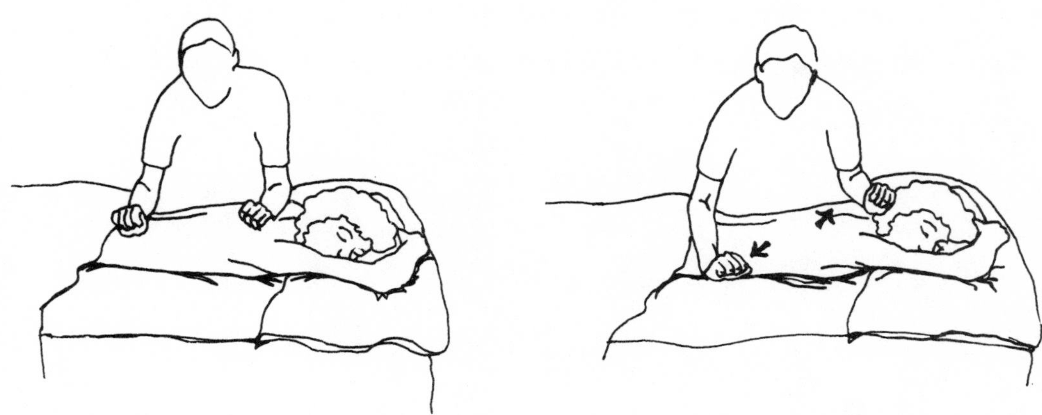

Big X

Lean your forearms close together across the center of your friend's back, make fists, and tilt your hands back so that the skin on the underside of your forearms is taut. Press hard and spread your forearms apart until they reach opposite ends of the spine. Now lift and return them to the middle of the back. You can make an X with this stroke by spreading your forearms to opposite hips and shoulders.

Main Stroke

Repeat the Main Stroke, with which you began, with this variation. Sitting or standing, at your friend's hips, begin the stroke with the heels of your hands resting on your friend's waist. Your fingertips are turned toward each other and placed on either side of the spine. Slide your palms in this position all the way to the shoulders. To return, hold either side of your friend's torso in your palms, and glide both hands down to the hips.

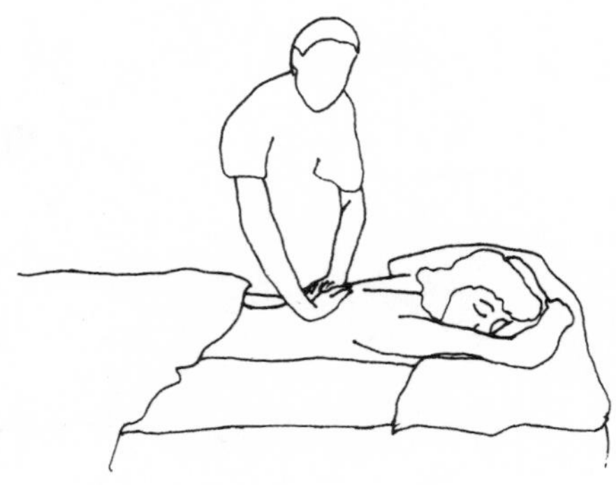

Press in and pull down slightly as you go. On the last upstroke, conclude the massage by gliding over the shoulders onto the upper arms. Slide your hands down both arms at once. Glide over your friend's palms and off the fingertips in a light, sweeping motion.

Palm on Palm

You can end this back rub with a "palm sandwich." Slide one of your hands under your friend's resting hand, and place your other palm over it. Your friend's hand will be lying between your palms. Hold this position lightly for about ten seconds. Then repeat with the other hand. Your friend's palms will be warm from the cradling.

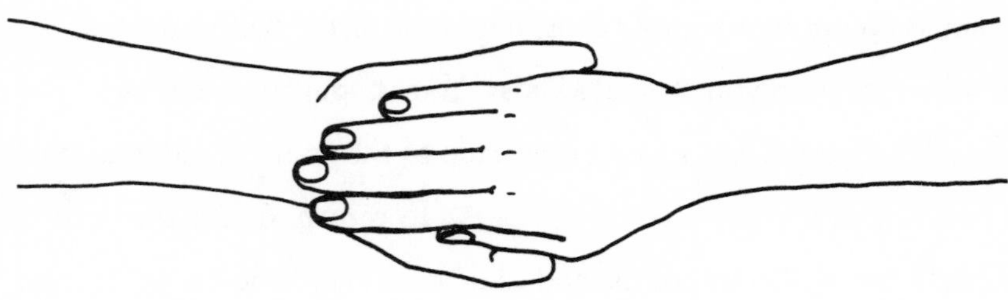

A VALENTINE BACK RUB

Sweet Somethings

A back rub is best when it comes from the heart. And "Let me give you a back rub" are lovely words in the language of love. Give your lover a delightful back massage for Valentine's Day.

You may have some questions in your mind about back rubs for lovers. What could you possibly do to a back that's sexy? you might ask. Or, how is an erotic back rub different from a friendly one? And, Why give a massage to my lover? We already touch while we're making love.

Diamonds Are Forever, but a Back Rub Is for Right Now

Any body part can become eroticized if it is treated with sensuality, interest, and care. Without any prior special interest in my feet as erotic objects, I chanced upon a man who taught me a lot about what you can do with toes. But that's another book. Back to the back.

The Back Is an Erotic Zone Worth Exploring

Some areas of the back that can be especially sensual are the back of the neck, especially the spot where it joins the back; the sides of the neck, especially the curve where the neck muscles move into the back; don't forget the armpits; the sides of the waist; the hips; the backside; the sacrum, at the lower back; the smoothness of the large area of skin of the whole back. I'm sure you can think of pleasant things to do to these areas of your lover's back, but to inspire you further, I've covered some interesting ways in the following back rub.

What individuals think is sexy or erotic varies a great deal. Some people assume that just because massage involves touching, it must be sexual, but that's not automatically so. Saying massage is always about sex is like saying travel is always about transportation. Massage is a language of touch that has many moods.

Sex and Backaches

Backaches have a reputation for being a popular form of birth control. Even though "Oh, my aching back!" is used as an excuse for not wanting to make love, all too often the backache is real. It's not much fun to make love when you're feeling sick or in pain. A back rub can be the perfect solution. You can satisfy some of your desire for physical communication with your lover through massage. And if he or she is in pain, you'll be giving a healing treatment. If the backache is not severe, and your back rub is terrific, maybe your lover's mood will improve along with the back, and desire will rear its delightful head.

Communication and Caring

You can communicate with your hands as wide a variety of things as you can say with your voice. Through touch you can communicate nurturing to a child, sympathy to a bereaved relative, affection to a good friend or family member, or eroticism to a lover. Massage can express all these feelings of caring.

When you give a massage to a lover with whom you already share physical intimacy, you can expand the scope of your physical communication. This will also increase your emotional communication. You can learn through massage new ways your lover likes to be touched. You may use the massage as part of extended foreplay. You can revive a tired lover. Or put to sleep an exhausted one.

You can show your caring for your lover through massage at times when other avenues of affection are not comfortable. Massage is a way to give a lover a great luxury when you might not be able to afford to buy one. Massage is a means to show your lover you care in ways that money can't buy. You might give a back rub just because you appreciate your lover's body. You may give a massage just because you want your lover to feel good.

The Erotic Back Rub

The distinction between a friendly back rub and a romantic one is a thin line, but we all know it when we feel it. The difference has more to do with how the stroke is done rather than which stroke is done.

An erotic massage is given to arouse rather than to calm the receiver. The following list describes some of the ways to alter strokes to heighten their eroticism:

Extremes of various kinds tend to be erotic. Very slow rhythms on a stroke that would otherwise feel "friendly" or therapeutic can make the stroke feel sensual. Sometimes a stroke done very quickly has a similar effect.

Extremes of pressure can be erotic. Slowly increasing pressure can feel wonderful on an area such as the sacrum. And extremely light stroking arouses most people in a pleasant way.

Rhythm plays a central part in sensuality, and you can experiment with it in massage.

Overlapping motions that produce a sensation of continuous, rhythmic movement tend to feel sensual. Strokes such as the Overlapping Palms on the thighs and the Waterfall on the spine are good examples. Circular strokes, such as Palm and Sole Circles, produce a slightly dizzying sensual effect.

Both the giver and the receiver being nude contributes to the mood.

Catering to a loved one's every desire is always seductive. A massage is a good way to express this mood. You can have fun with inventing personal ways of tailoring the massage to your lover's tastes.

Isn't it your turn to receive a back rub?

For Your Valentine

One hour

Main Stroke—2 sets down whole back of body

Palm Circles—8 palms & soles together
4 both palms
4 sacrum
8 sacrum & back of neck together

Main Stroke—1 lower back to shoulders

Trapezius Laps—8 each shoulder

Rocking Horse—1 down spine

Waterfall—2 up & down

Cupid's Arrow: Outlining the Sacrum—1

Buttock Circles—8

Thigh Pockets—8 each thigh

Thigh Waves—2 down & up

Main Stroke—1 buttocks to shoulders & down

Braiding—2 down & up & down

Main Stroke—1 hips to feet; 1 whole back of body

Back of Knee & Elbow Circles—4 simultaneous

Feet Squeeze—4 together

Main Stroke with Arms—1

Palm & Sole Circles—4 alternating pairs

Palm Circles—5 both palms

Palm Feathers—1 both palms

Short But Sweet Valentine Back Rub

½ hour

♡ **Marks short back rub strokes**

Main Stroke—2 sets down whole back of body

Palm Circles—8 both palms

Rocking Horse—1

Waterfall—2

Cupid's Arrow: Outlining the Sacrum—1

Buttock Circles—4

Thigh Waves—2

Braiding—2

Main Stroke—1 down whole back of body

Feet Squeeze—2

Palm & Sole Circles—4

Palm Feathers—2 both palms

FOR YOUR VALENTINE

As in other areas with lovers, we are generous with a back rub. We define the back as the whole back of the body. Use your imagination and a lightly scented oil.

Main Stroke: Whole Back of Body ♡

Stand above your lover's head and rest your palms on his or her shoulders. Your fingers are pointing toward the spine but are not on it. Lean forward onto your hands to achieve firm pressure; press harder with your fingertips. Slide your hands down the muscles of the back to either side of the spine. When your hands cross the buttocks, walk to one side and pivot your palms so the heels are on the outer edges of either thigh and the fingers are pointing toward each other resting on the inner thighs. You are

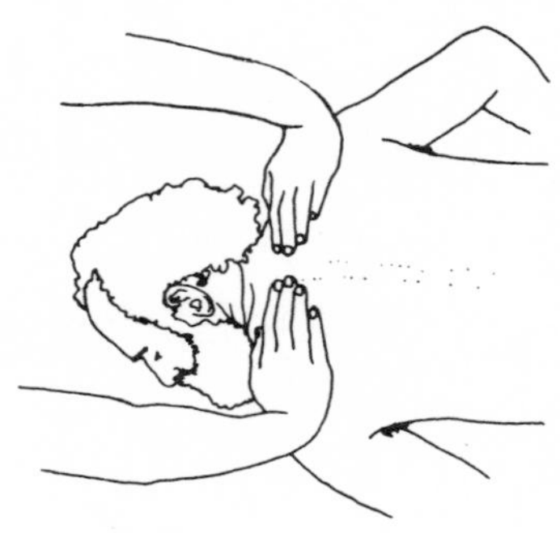

now facing your lover's head. From this position you can continue the Main Stroke all the way down the legs to the feet.

Now return up the whole back of the body. With a palm on each ankle, press and slide your hands up both legs, over the hips, and up the back to the shoulders. Cover the whole back of the body with this stroke.

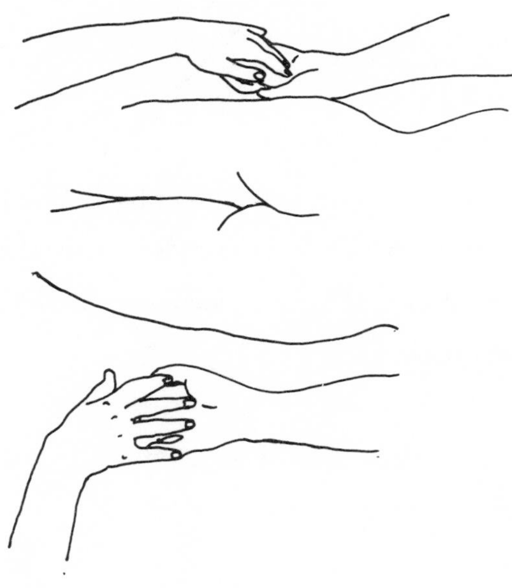

Palm Circles ♡

This is a simple and very pleasant stroke. Stand or sit to one side of your lover. Her or his arms should be at their sides with the palms up. Place the fingertips of one hand in one of your lover's palms. Place the fingertips of your other hand in the arch of your lover's foot nearest you. Make gentle but firm circles with both your hands in these spots simultaneously. Next move one of your hands to your lover's other hand and make simultaneous circles in both palms. Keep one hand on your lover's

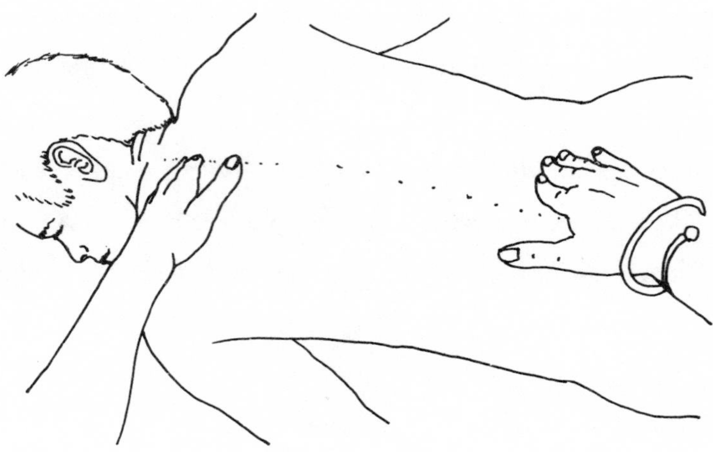

palm and move your other hand to the lower back. Use both your hands to make circles in these two spots. Now move the hand in the palm to the back of your lover's neck and make simultaneous circles on the upper spine and the lower back.

Main Stroke

Bring both your hands to the lower back and do the Main Stroke up the back muscles to the shoulders.

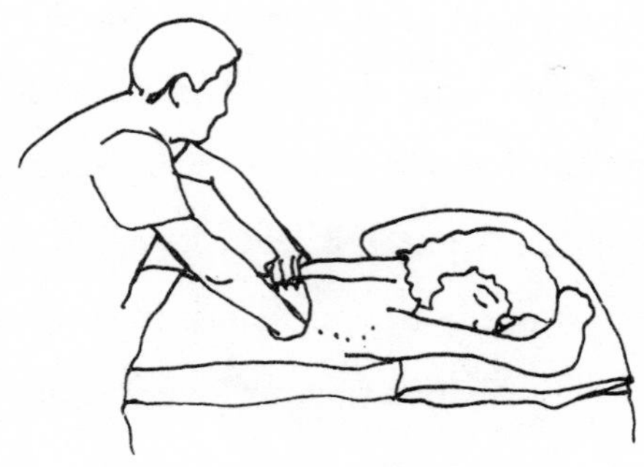

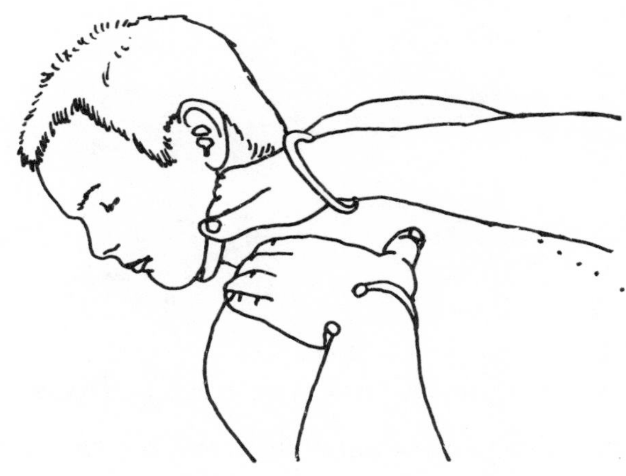

Trapezius Laps

Standing or sitting to one side of your lover's back, place your fingertips on the muscles to one side of the neck. Press and slide one hand up from the shoulder muscle slightly onto the muscles of the upper back. As the fingertips of this hand reach the area between the shoulder blades, begin drawing your other hand up the neck and shoulder muscles across the same area. Continue this double hand motion back and forth across the trapezius muscle, from the neck to the outer edge of the shoulder. It is most wonderful when your strokes overlap and the motion feels continuous.

Rocking Horse ♡

Standing or sitting near your lover's right hip, place your right palm on the sacrum, fingers pointing toward the head. Cross and cover this hand with your left palm, fingers pointing toward you. Slide your two hands as a

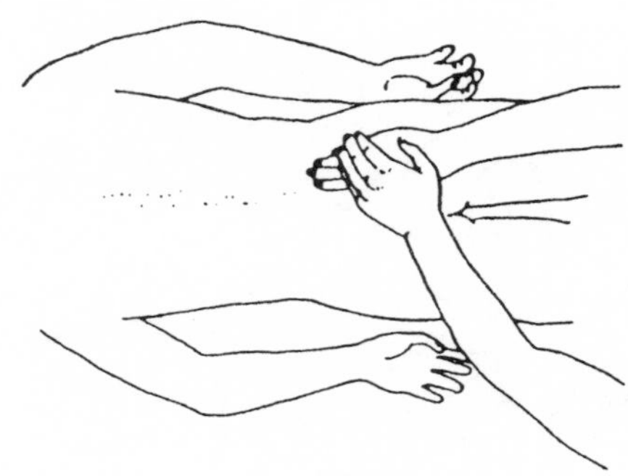

unit up the spine, keeping a steady, moderate pressure. (Never press down hard directly on the spine.) At the top of the spine, reverse the motion and draw your hands to the waist again. Dig the tips of each forefinger and middle finger into the grooves on either side of the spine. Press harder than on the way up. When you reach the sacrum, move up the spine again with your flat palm. This stroke's name comes from the rocking motion you achieve if the up and down strokes are done continuously.

Waterfall ♡

Begin at the top of the spine with the tips of the first two fingers of your right hand pressing into the muscles on either side of the vertebrae. Slide your fingertips two or three inches down the muscles on either side of the

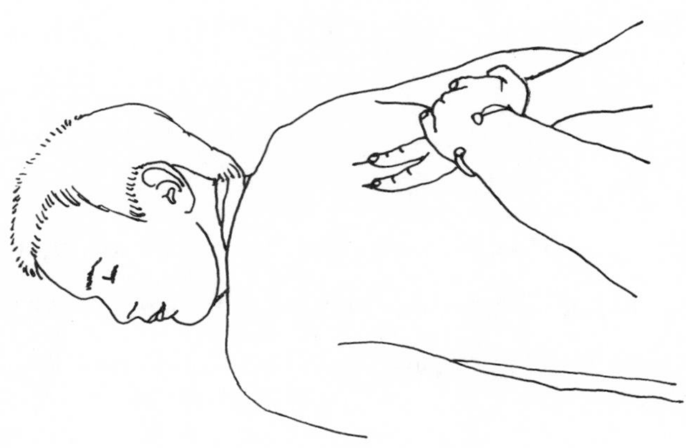

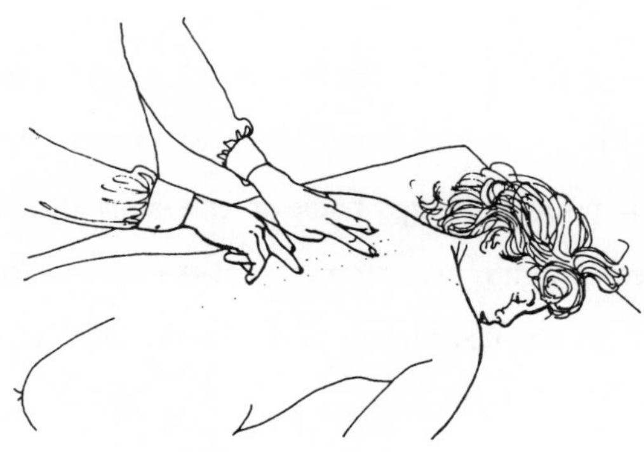

spine. Then begin the same pressing, sliding motion with the first two fingertips of your left hand, covering the area your right hand has just covered. Lift your right hand and slide the fingers of your left hand an inch or so farther down the back. Now lift your left hand and slide the fingertips of your right hand a few inches farther down the back. Keep repeating this alternating sliding and pressing with your fingertips on both sides of the spine. As one pair of fingertips is pressing, raise the other off the back. Then start the motion with your other hand. On the receiving end the stroke correctly done will feel like a waterfall or having something smooth roll down the back.

Cupid's Arrow: Outlining the Sacrum ♡

Bring your hands to the lower spine. The sacrum is a flat bone at the base of the spine, shaped like an arrowhead pointing to the feet. With your fingertips, press and trace the outline of the sacrum by moving them away

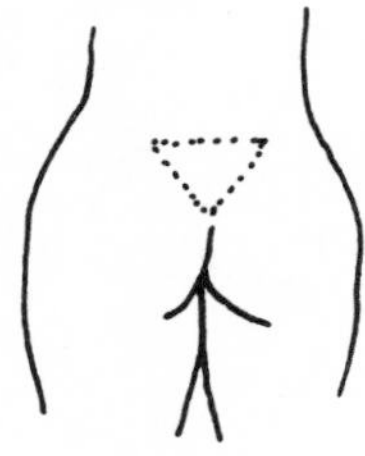

from either side of the spine at the top of the sacrum, to the tips, and down the sides to the coccyx or tailbone. When you reach the tip, reverse the motion and slide your fingertips back up the sides and across the top, until they come together again on either side of the spine. You can add several overlapping thumb strokes on top of the arrow bone as you finish.

Buttock Circles ♡

The muscles of the hips and buttocks endure much pressure during the day from sitting and standing and can use some deep pressure massage. Stand or kneel just below the level of your lover's hips, resting your body weight on your palms and pressing into the muscles. Make large circles on the buttocks with the palms of your hands. Slide your hands up across the hips from the "sitting bones" so that your palms are massaging the muscles. Now rotate your fingertips out over the hipbones and down the outside of the hips. Bring the heels of your hands back to the beginning position under the sitting bones, slightly lifting the buttocks. Repeat this stroke in a continuous, circular pattern.

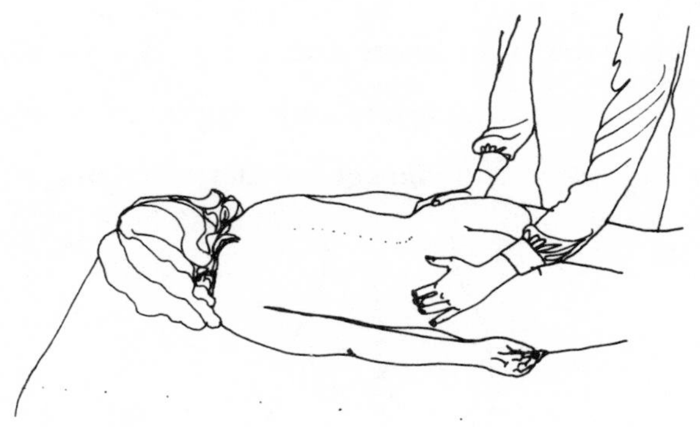

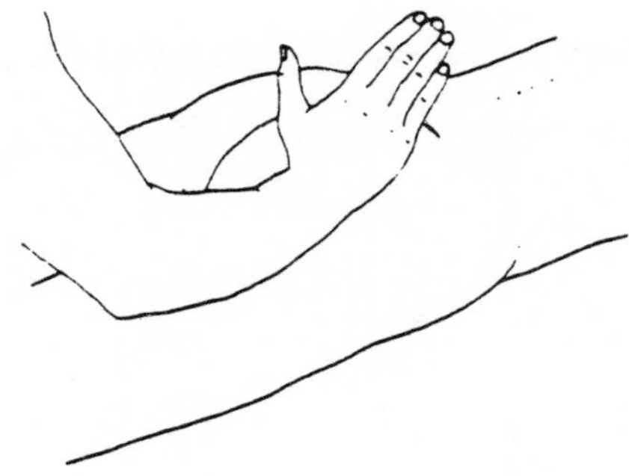

Thigh Pockets

This stroke is done with the heels of your hands in overlapping, upward motion. Find the depressions to either side of both sitting bones. Place a palm over one pocket and press in while sliding the heel of your hand up the buttock. Begin the same motion with your other hand over the same area just as you are reaching the top of the buttock with the first hand. This stroke has a pleasant, kneading motion when done rhythmically and is quite soothing to the lower back and legs. Repeat on the other leg.

Thigh Waves ♡

On the inside of the thigh just above the knee, draw your hands upward in slow, hand-over-hand strokes. Begin a new hand slide just as you are

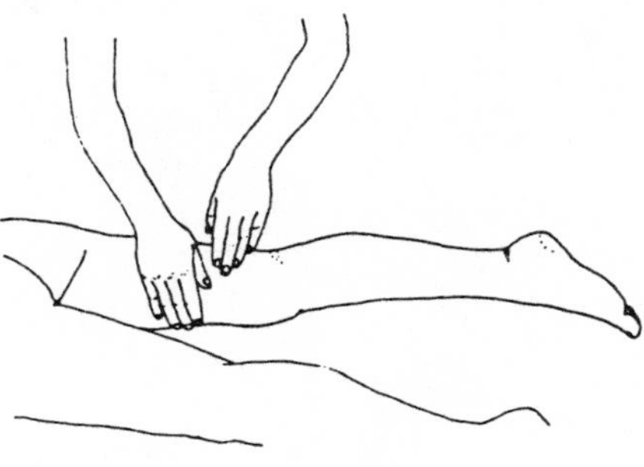

finishing the previous one. The pressure is gentle, the rhythm steady, and the palms stay in contact with the skin. Move up the leg as you go, to the crease between the leg and the buttock. Then repeat on the other thigh.

Main Stroke

Repeat the Main Stroke once from the buttocks to the shoulders and back again.

Braiding ♡

Use your palms to make a braiding motion on the back. Begin with the heels of your hands resting on the bed to either side of the upper back. Move your fingertips toward each other, toward the spine. Just before they touch, move your hands slightly away from each other so that they can continue all the way down your lover's sides again to the bed. Now reverse the motion: slide the heels of your hands across the spine and pivot your fingertips to the bed. Your forearms will make an X as they cross. Repeat this crossover stroking up and down from the shoulders to the hips.

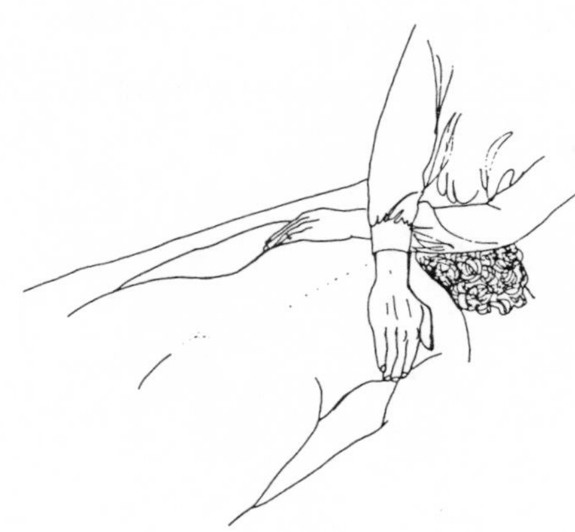

Main Stroke ♡

As your reach the hips after braiding, begin the Main Stroke down the legs to the feet. Then return to the shoulders with the Main Stroke, and continue back down the whole length of the body to the feet.

Back of Knee & Elbow Circles

Use a circular stroking with your fingertips on the backs of the knees and elbows. Try circling one hand on the back of one knee while circling the other hand in the crook of the arm. Then circle the opposite elbow and knee areas.

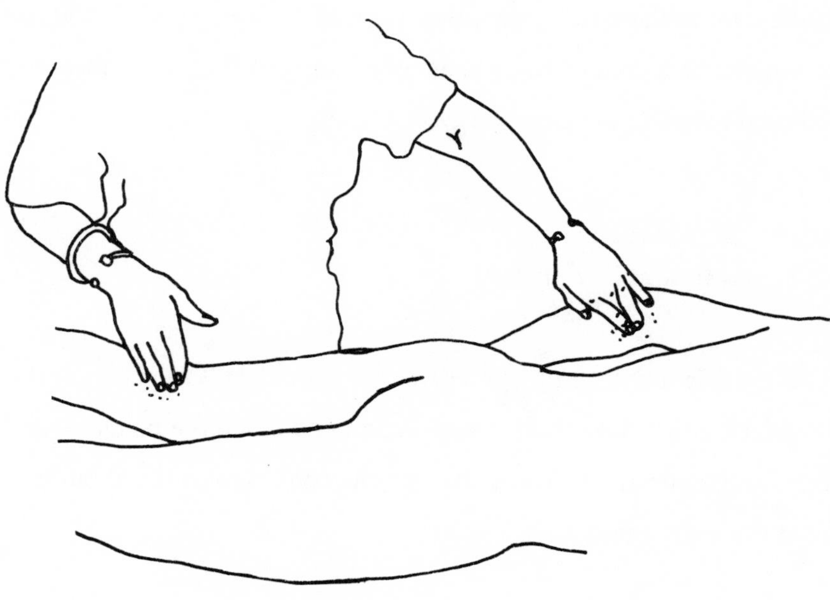

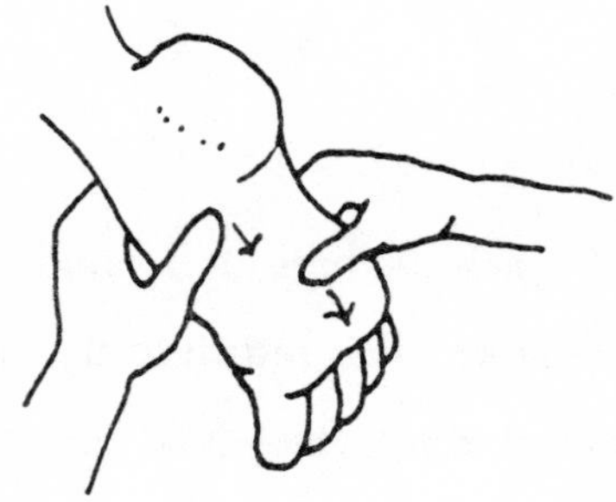

Feet Squeeze ♡

Use more oil on the feet for this stroke than you normally would. Pick up the left foot with both your hands. Have your thumbs on the sole of the foot and the rest of your fingers on the top. Move your hands in an overlapping, squeezing motion. Start with your left thumb at the base of the heel. Squeeze the foot with your left hand and drag your hand down the foot to the base of the toes. Press hard with your thumb. Just before your left thumb reaches the base of the toes, begin the same squeezing and dragging with your right thumb. Now pick up your left hand and start the stroke over at the base of the heel. Try it at different speeds. You can also massage both feet at once by using one hand per foot and squeezing and pulling downward simultaneously.

Main Stroke with Arms

Do the Main Stroke up the legs to the shoulders. On reaching the shoulders, come down both arms. When you reach the palms, slide both your hands onto the hips and then up the back, across the shoulders, and down the arms again.

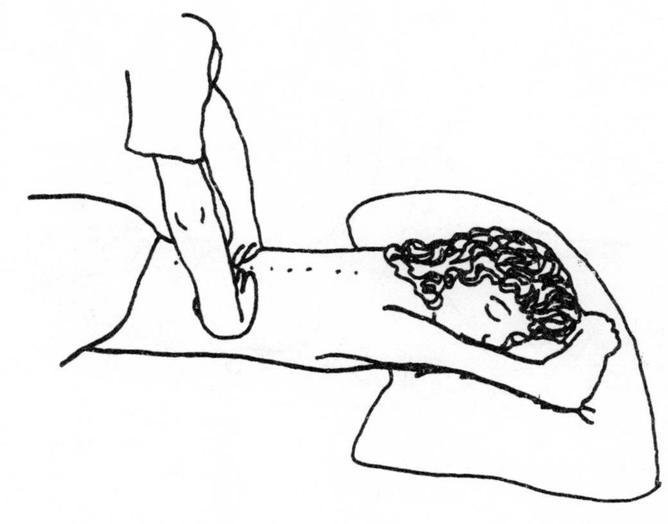

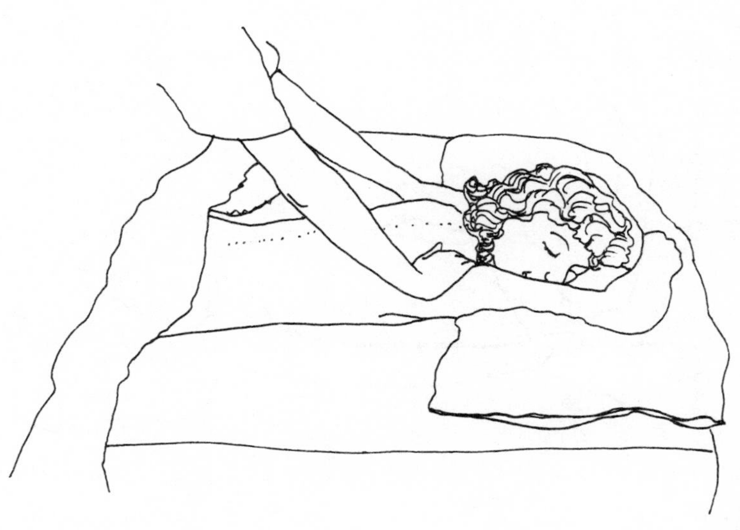

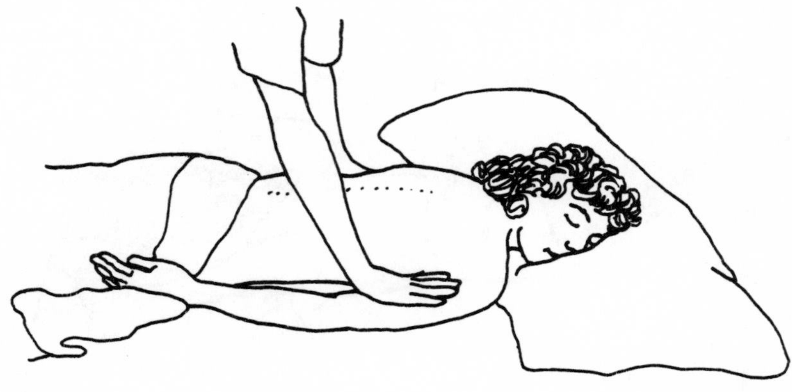

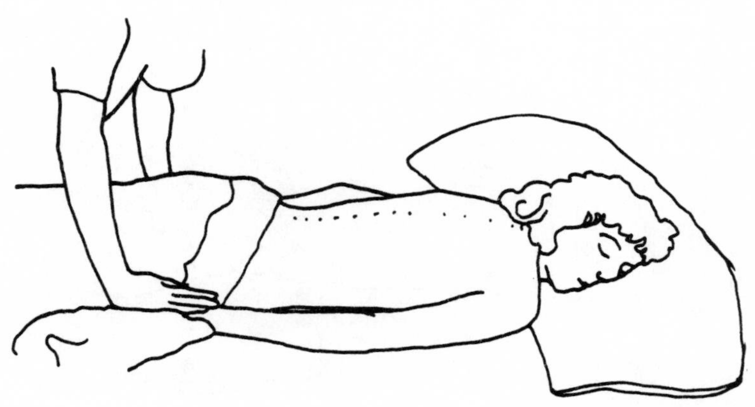

Palm & Sole Circles ♡

Make circles with your fingertips in the palm of one hand and the arch of one foot. Then do the same on the other palm and foot. Try also circling in opposite palms and feet.

Palm Circles

Make slow circles with your fingertips on both palms at once.

Palm Feathers ♡

Using your fingertips with very light pressure, glide your hands across your lover's palms, down the length of the fingers, and off the fingertips. Repeat this stroking motion several times as a tantalizing finale to your grand Valentine Back Rub.

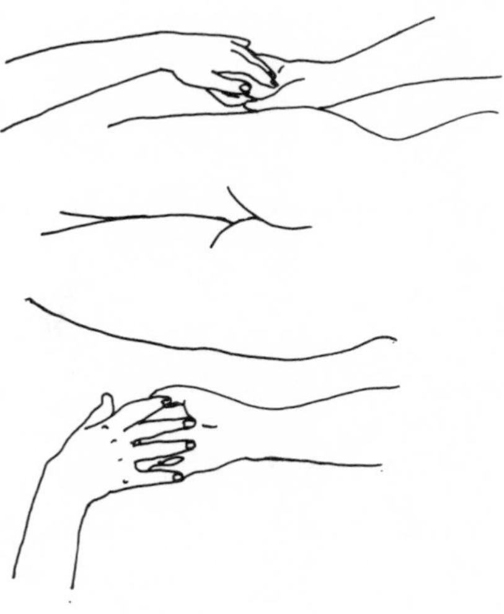

Special Occasions Fit For a Back Rub

Birthday

Anniversary

Christmas

New Year

Valentine's Day

Bastille Day

Labor Day

Thanksgiving

Mother's Day

Father's Day

Grandmother's Day

Grandfather's Day

Graduation

Morning After

Blue Monday (Tuesday, Wednesday . . .)

Just Got a Raise

Just Been Hired

Just Been Fired

Won the Lottery

Just Moved

Unbirthday

Bedtime

Teatime

Anytime

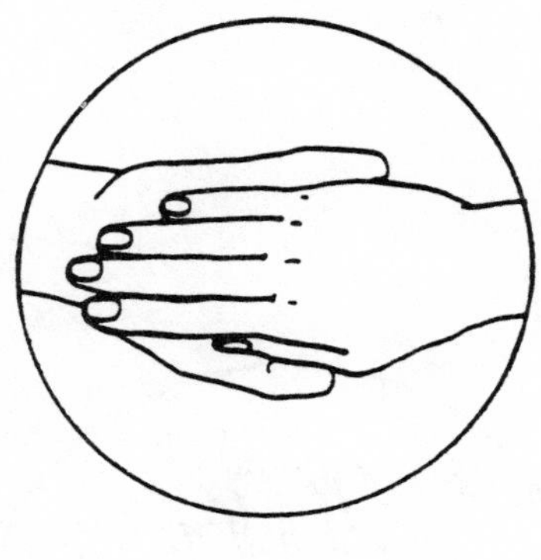

HEALING

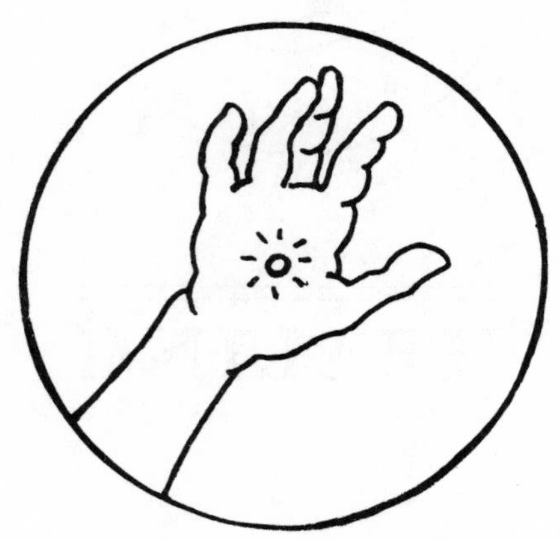

THE BACK RUB PERSONALITY

Psychological associations with body parts are rooted in the parts' functions. The back bears burdens and thus is associated with a person's sense of limits and capacities for work or stress. A "backache personality" is often recognizable as overambitious or strongly prone to placing mind over matter. "Spineless," "no backbone," or "backing out" are phrases used about people we feel have shirked their rightful burdens.

Aim for a "back rub personality" rather than a "backache personality." If you think you have a back problem that is caused largely by stress rather than physical trauma, it is still a priority to treat the physical symptom first. Often when the physical symptom of a back problem is taken care of, the psychological problem surfaces. You can't ignore your body and function well. The body is one of your natural limits. If you respect a limit, it becomes a resource.

YOUR NATURAL RHYTHM

Rhythm is an aspect of a person's metabolism to which others often have strong reactions. You can like or dislike someone because he or she is speedy or slow paced, erratic or consistent. The breath is at the core of this body rhythm, and like snowflakes, each person has a unique natural breathing pattern. If you learn to recognize your rhythm, you can broaden your insight into your moods, gain more control over your physical states, and increase your ability to minimize stress.

Moods and Breathing

Notice that when you are excited you breathe relatively fast and high in your chest. Holding your breath is a sign of tense anticipation. Slow breathing is an aspect of relaxation and calm. Deep breathing is an aspect of deep emotion. Most of the time we let our breathing rhythms occur unconsciously, without being aware of how much they affect our moods.

If you reverse this process and change your breathing rhythm consciously from time to time, you'll find you can alter your emotional states considerably. Knowledge of breathing is a useful relaxation skill because you can implement it in any situation, without needing privacy, equipment, or extra time. You can give yourself an inner back rub.

How to Find Your Basic Breath

First you need to learn to find the natural breathing rhythm you would have if no outside influences interfered. The Basic Breath exercise that follows teaches you how to do this. Once you have a sense of your own relaxed rhythm, you have a middle point from which to gauge variations in a spectrum from very tense to very relaxed. Any time you want to relax, it's simple to do the Basic Breath and improve your state.

The Basic Breath can be used for healing—to increase circulation in an area, to speed up tissue regeneration after injury, to relieve the pain of headaches and backaches.

The Basic Breath exercise was developed by Magdalene Proskauer, a San Francisco therapist who specializes in analyzing the psychological aspects of breathing.

THE BASIC BREATH

There are different Proskauer exercises for each part of the body, but the same three-part breath is used in all of them. This breathing cycle is designed to trigger your natural rhythm gradually. By using this cycle you can let go of imposed rhythms and allow your own to surface.

Lie on your back on the bed or floor. Relax your arms at your sides and let your feet fall out to the sides. Close your eyes and feel the way you are lying on the floor. Notice whether any part of your body feels a bit tense or doesn't seem to be resting comfortably on the surface beneath you. Now move your focus inside your body and notice where you feel movement as you breathe.

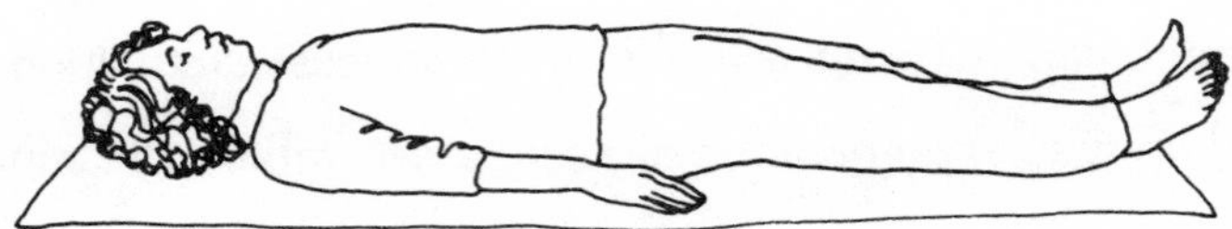

If you feel tense anywhere, try imagining that you can breathe into the tension, as though you could actually exhale through that body part. Imagine the breath relaxing your sore muscle as it moves through it. Breathing into a body part is something you can do anywhere, any time you feel tense or nervous. Locate the tight place and "breathe into it." Breathe in sync with the tensing (inhale) and relaxing (exhale) of your movement.

As you are doing this exercise, loosen your clothing if it is tight at the waist. Let the muscles of your stomach and abdomen relax and let your breath sink lower in your body. Place one hand palm down at the lowest place on your torso where you can feel the motion of your breathing. Let your hand rest on this place awhile until you begin to feel the rise and fall of your body under your palm from your breathing. Now let your hand and arm relax at your side again. If you see any pictures of yourself or other images during this breathing exercise, remember them and draw or write them down later.

Relax your jaw and open your mouth a little so that you can exhale through your mouth. You don't need to breathe heavily. Relax and breathe naturally. Inhale through your nose; exhale through your mouth; and pause at the end of the exhalation before you breathe again.

This pause is the key to the effectiveness of the breathing. Crucial things are happening to your body during the pause; you are actually still exhaling, though you may feel as though nothing is going on. Deepening your exhalation gets all the stale air out of your lungs, and makes more room for fresh air when you inhale. Most of us don't exhale deeply enough. Often, when you feel that you can't take in enough air, and that you'd like to inhale more deeply, it's because you haven't exhaled fully enough to make room in your lungs for new air. This is usually the breathing difficulty in asthma. Lengthening your exhalation can help release asthmatic symptoms.

You have paused at the end of the exhalation for a long time now. Let yourself really explore the pause. How does it feel to you? Does it feel too long? Not long enough? Are you a little worried that your body won't breathe in again unless you make it? Think of your breathing when you are asleep. You don't have to tell yourself to breathe then. Think of animals breathing when they are resting. Their breath is long and rolling. They don't tell themselves to breathe. You can learn to trust that your breath will always come in again.

Allow the pause to be as long as it wants. It may feel very long. See whether you can wait and stay with the pause until your body wants to breathe in again by itself. Inhale through your nose; exhale through your mouth; then pause and wait. It's a little like standing on the beach and waiting for another wave to come in. Try to find a pace at which you are

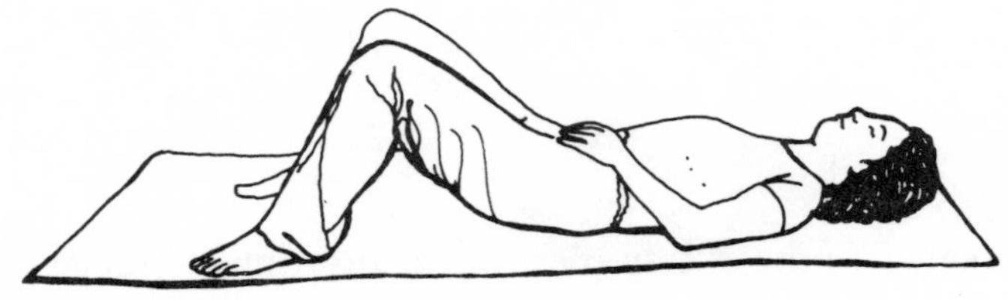

neither holding your breath to prolong the pause nor making yourself breathe in again. Let yourself breathe in this pattern as long as you want.

This exercise in itself is deeply relaxing. If you have difficulty going to sleep, you can use this breath at night. Or any time you feel tense you can take a few minutes off for yourself, relax, and find your rhythm again. The Basic Breath is a gentle, powerful, centering exercise.

Breathing Away Pain

Now that you know the Basic Breath, you can apply it to pain relief. As you imagine you are breathing into a body part, you stimulate circulation in that area. More blood flows to the painful spot, warming it, bringing more oxygen to decrease aching, carrying away waste materials from the cells, and generally reviving and relaxing the tissue. What you usually sense as a result of breathing into the body part is a warming and softening of the muscle and sometimes a tingling sensation from the change in circulation. This relaxation of the tissue will immediately cause some relief of your aches and pains. For relief of severe pain, continue the breathing process longer. No body part is unreachable by the breath.

Adding a small movement to your breathing exercise can also increase its effectiveness at relieving pain. Although you need not be in any particular position, the quickest pain relief comes from doing the exercise while lying down because you can give over the work of holding up your weight to the bed or floor and put all your attention on relaxing.

In general, you want to make very tiny movements of the sore body part. Synchronize the motions with your breathing. Inhale as you lift or stretch. Exhale as you release or bend. Most tension release occurs on the exhalation, as you "let go" with your muscles.

BREATH MASSAGE

The therapist Magdalene Proskauer has developed a technique of touch coordinated with breathing that encourages the receiver to release deep muscle tension. A simple version of this technique can be done for back tension.

Eyes closed, your friend is lying down in a comfortable position on his or her stomach. Stand or sit beside your friend near the waist. Watch the surface of the back as your friend breathes and note where the back muscles are moving as a result of the breathing. Lightly place your fingertips on the highest (most near the shoulders) area where you see movement. As your friend exhales, draw your fingertips down the back a few inches. Use an extremely light touch that might be the smooth brush of a feather—or the breath—across the muscle. Stroke only on the exhalation.

At the end of the exhalation, pause with your fingertips lightly on the back and wait there as your friend inhales. As the next exhalation begins, draw your feather touch another short distance lower. Take your time and allow your touch to guide your friend's breathing deeper into his or her body. Continue this pattern until you can see that the breath has reached the pelvic area by slight movement of the muscles in the lower back. Lightly move your hands away from the body.

This subtle technique is deceptively simple. If it is done well, your friend will feel as though their muscles have been massaged from the inside. Breath massage is extremely calming, and it is particularly useful for anyone who is bedridden or sore and might be unable to enjoy being massaged with a deeper touch.

VISUALIZATION

Visualization in the realm of healing means using healthy images of your body to improve your physical condition. There are two steps in the process. For example, if you have a slipped disk, allow yourself to see an image in your mind's eye of the current state of that body part, imaging what the disk looks like—out of place and inflamed. Next, visualize the disk where it should be. Looking at anatomy charts is useful. Throughout the day bring this healthy picture of your well-aligned spine to mind to encourage healing.

Body Images

This mental process is an ancient technique, which shamans, yogis, and witches have used throughout history. Many Western medical doctors now use visualization effectively to help cancer patients and injured athletes. Sports medicine often incorporates excellent, unusual treatments earlier than other branches of medicine. Visualization is useful for people who are in pain, too tired, or just too sick to do other kinds of treatment or exercise. You can also try encouraging healing in other people by visualizing them healthy.

Athletes often use visualization as part of their warm-up routines. Visualize yourself doing an exercise or sport before the event. Imagining something stimulates many of the same responses in your nerves and muscles as actually doing it. Visualization can be used as a form of practice that will improve your performance. You can also use visualization as a preventive technique by maintaining a healthy image of your body in top shape throughout the day.

Waking Dreams

Visualization is a powerful tool in emotional healing. Our dreams and fantasies are pictures of our emotional states. Look to your dream images for information about your deep feelings. Practice waking dreams; that is, visualize your feelings and actions in new, desirable ways to expand your self-image.

People tend to have either literal or conceptual visions. If two people are using visualization to heal shinsplints, the conceptual visionary might see a horse running free in a sunny field. The literal visionary would see a healed shinbone.

AN INNER BACK RUB

Visualization can be used to explore internally an emotional or physical pain. Imagine you can shrink yourself and walk into your body to search and do internal maintenance. Don't preplan the story; simply try to let the events occur. They will.

Lie down, close your eyes, and relax your breathing. If you have a specific ache or pain you want to work on, locate it and then choose a natural body opening as your "entrance way." Imagine you can shrink yourself or someone else to about a half inch or smaller.

The journey in and out is just as important as the destination. Resist hurrying or missing any steps. You can talk out loud about what you are doing and how it feels to you. If you have a pain in your upper back you want to reach, you could enter through your mouth. Look around at the setting and describe it. "I am walking up to the mouth. I am crawling over the lips. As I let myself down inside, the surface becomes slippery. It's dark in here. I'm walking toward the back of the mouth on the teeth. They feel sharp and bumpy."

When you reach the back of the mouth, decide how to get down the throat and into the shoulder. "There's a deep hole here like a well. There's no way to get down except jump, but I don't know where I'll land." You can decide to go on or try another way. "I think I'll just jump." Describe your descent, what you see, how you feel. Almost always a surprise landing takes place; if not, pick something to catch onto to stop yourself when you feel you've fallen far enough.

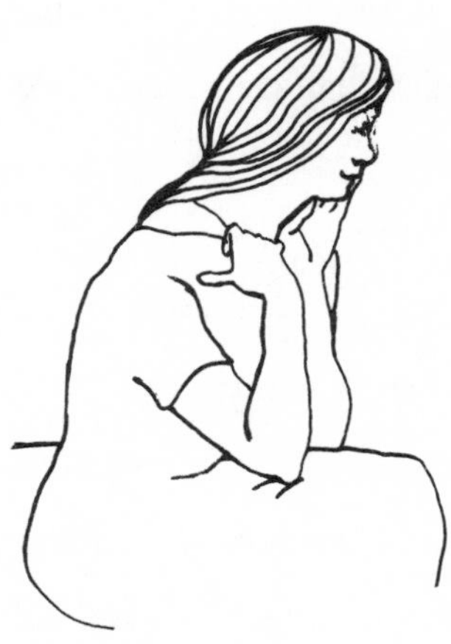

When you land, decide how you're going to get to your sore muscle. You can swim through an artery or walk along a tendon. When you reach the sore muscle, look around. Describe what you see. Try to imagine a way you could massage the muscle by walking on it or squeezing it. Imagine you are doing this. Take your time.

When you have massaged to your satisfaction, begin your journey out of the body. Out again, imagine you can expand to your normal size and merge with your larger body again. Take a moment to check how the previously sore muscle feels now. Often it feels greatly relaxed!

STRESS REDUCTION

With stress, it's the little things that mean a lot. The conclusion of a study on stress conducted by Richard Lazarus and colleagues at the University of California, Berkeley, is that relatively minor yet frequent annoyances have a more destructive effect on our health than do grand-scale traumas.

A Back Rub a Day Keeps the Doctor Away

The good news is that small tension relief sessions performed frequently throughout the day can have a big effect on relieving stress. Make healing a way of life. Include short stretching and breathing breaks in each day's routine to keep the little stresses from snowballing. Exchange a brief session of shoulder massage with a co-worker. Take a moment to bend over in your chair and relax your back several times a day. Sprinkle back exercises throughout your daily routine. You'll be doing yourself a big preventive favor.

Raising Your Pleasure Quota

Another UC, Berkeley, study found that to be free of stress, it's not enough to eliminate negative factors from your life. You have to *add* positive ones. This is a program worth lots of attention.

Fill your life with treats, luxuries, and happy experiences. Lavish your loved ones with small signs of affection and big treats. Up your pleasure quota. Remember, massage is to stress as a bath is to a day's dirt. Get used to being good to yourself and others. Get more back rubs. Doctor's orders.

PRESSURE POINT MASSAGE

Shiatsu is a specialized method of finger pressure massage developed centuries ago in Japan and still practiced today. It is particularly good for tension relief because it enables the practitioner, novice or pro, to effect simple but deep physical release of tension. Shiatsu pressure points conform to the acupuncture map of energy centers and channels in our bodies. Pressure point treatment of acupuncture points creates a milder form of the very powerful healing relief of acupuncture.

Distinct from Swedish or Esalen style massage, pressure point massage is performed mainly by pressing your fingertips quite firmly and deeply into a single spot on a muscle. The key to doing it well is to apply and release pressure extremely gradually. No oil or other lubricant is used because you do not want your hands to slide. Classic shiatsu is a series of fingertip massages in specific patterns. However, you can use simple pressure point technique on many back muscles and achieve an unusually relaxing effect.

A Pressure Point Back Rub

20 minutes

Back of Head & Neck

Shoulder Points

Lower Back and Sacrum Points

Spine Points

Spine Sweep

A PRESSURE POINT BACK RUB

Back of Head and Neck

On all areas, apply and release pressure very gradually. You can ask your friend to tell you when to go deeper or lighten up. While your friend is lying on his or her back, use the fingertips of both your hands to press all over the back of the skull. Be thorough.

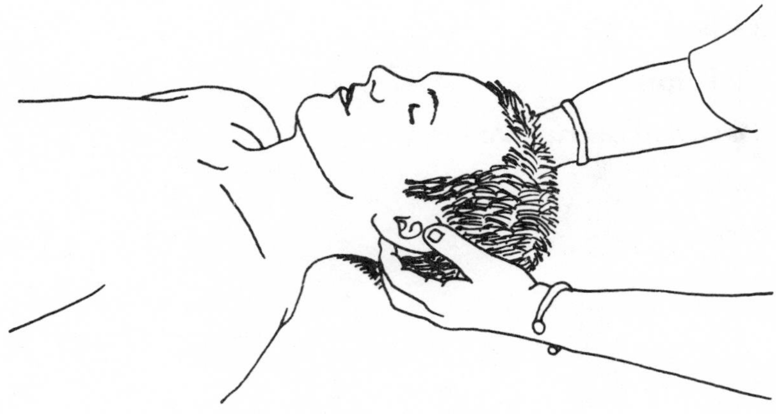

Now have your friend lie on his or her stomach. The occipital ridge is the concave area where the base of the skull meets the neck. Most of us collect much tension here. Linger on these points. Find "holes" as well as tight areas under the ridge. Press deeply with the thumb of one hand while bracing the head with your other hand to counteract the pressure.

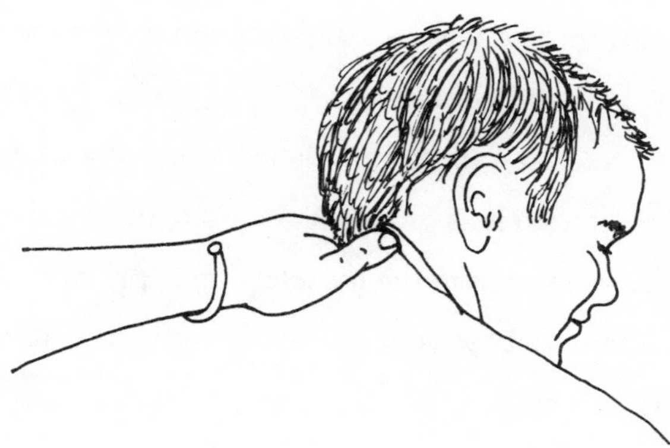

Place your thumbs on both sides of the cervical vertebrae at the base of the skull on the neck muscles that stretch from the occipital ridge down to the base of the neck as it enters the shoulders. Apply gradual pressure along the muscles. Give this treatment special attention and slow, gentle pressure.

Shoulder Points

Stand above your friend's head. Resting your palms lightly on either shoulder, use both thumbs to apply gradual pressure along the trapezius muscle, running from the neck to the outer edges of the shoulders. When

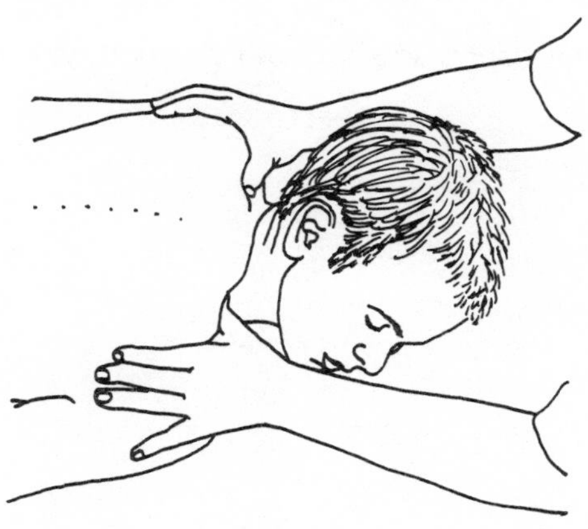

you find a spot on the muscle that feels tight, spend more time there to relieve the tension. Thumb pressure should be applied very gradually until you reach a level where you want to be still and hold for a while. When you release the pressure, do it as gradually as you applied it. Don't hurt your friend; this causes tension in the muscle. Apply pressure up to the point of soreness. Then wait for your friend's muscles to relax and soften and move on to the next spot.

Lower Back & Sacrum Points

Stand beside your friend's hips. Lean your weight into your arms as you press your thumbs on either side of the highest sacral vertebra. Gradually angle more of your weight into your hands. When you want to release the pressure, do it just as gradually as you applied it. Then move your thumbs down beside the next sacral vertebra. Apply the pressure of your body weight again. Work your way from the top of the sacrum to the tip. Then apply the same type of gradual pressure to the lower outsides of the sacrum, from the waist to the tailbone. The pressure should be deep but not painful to your friend. If it is painful, you are pressing either too quickly or too hard for her or him to relax with the pressure. You might not be in quite the right spot, so shift your position and try another spot.

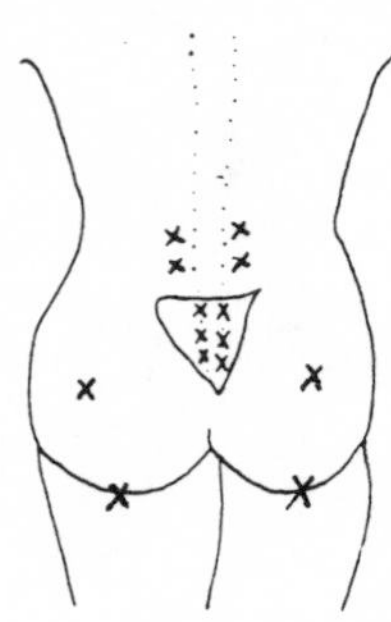

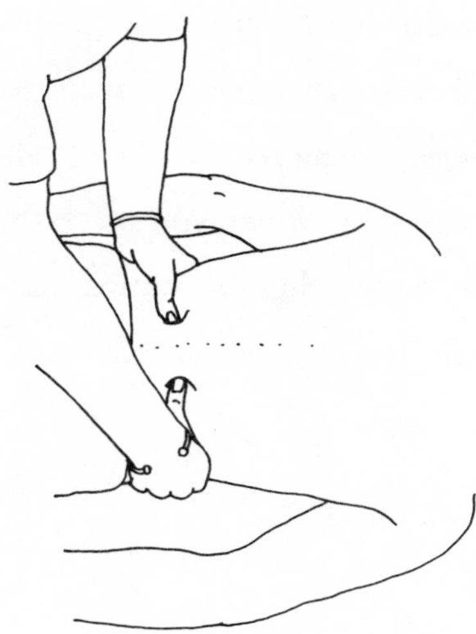

Spine Points

Place your thumbs on the muscles on either side of the top of the spine. Lean your weight firmly but gradually down onto your hands and angle your finger pressure slightly in toward the space between two vertebrae.

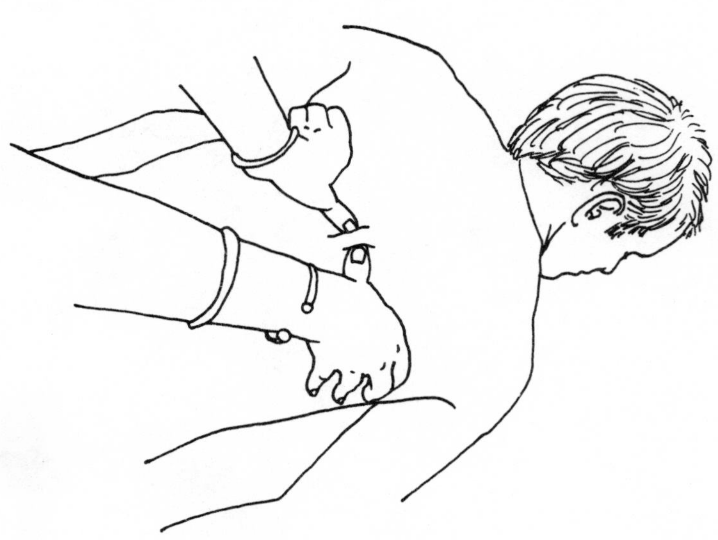

Hold this pressure a moment. Then release gradually and move your thumbs to between the next pair of vertebrae. Repeat this pressure and release between the vertebrae along the whole spinal column. Take care that you don't skip a vertebra. When you reach the waist area, just below the ribs, be sure to angle your thumbs toward each other. Do not press down on the spine at the curve of the back.

Spine Sweep

This stroke will connect the separate strokes you've done. Place your palms on your friend's shoulders as he or she is lying on the stomach. Draw your palms along the muscles on either side of the spine down the back and over the hips. As you cross the hips, angle your hands away and lift them off the body. Return your palms to the shoulders and begin the sweep again with light, swift strokes. Repeat six or eight times.

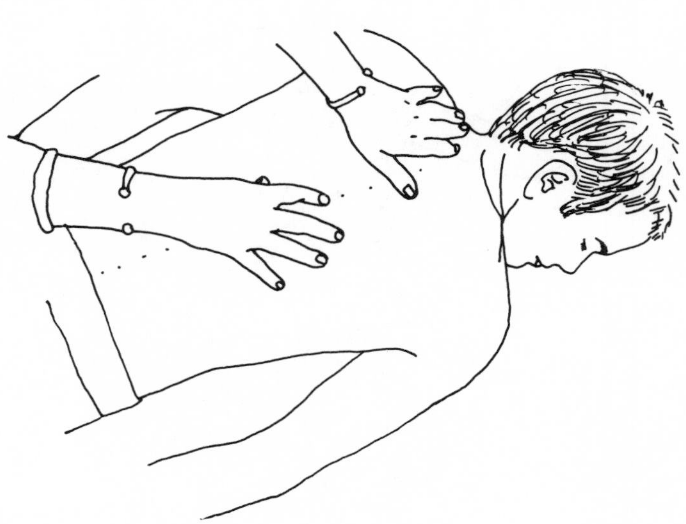

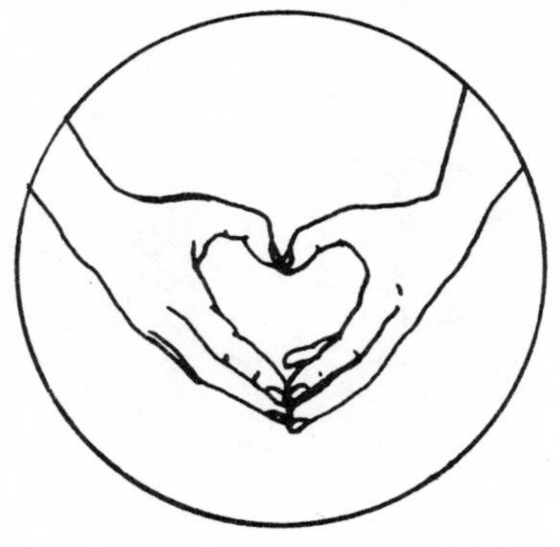

GOOD NIGHT & SWEET DREAMS

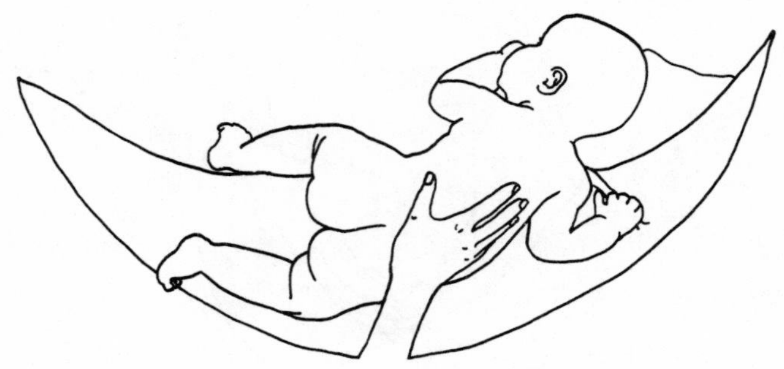

SLEEP CYCLES

Human metabolism cycles in hour and a half increments. If you note a particular time of day when you are especially sleepy (or especially wide awake), you can calculate your sleepy (and waking) cycles from this time.

For example, if you tend to wake up naturally in the morning at 6:45 AM, your next wide awake cycle will peak at 8:15AM, an hour and a half later. On this schedule, your sleepy cycles would fall at 7:30 AM, then 9:00 AM, then 10:30 AM, and so on. If you know this, you'll know that you'll have an easier time getting up at 6:45 than you will at 7:30. You also might note that you'll be due for a sleepy cycle peak at noon; try to schedule lunch meetings at 12:30 rather than 12:00 so you'll be moving toward a peak of one of your waking cycles.

Figuring these cycles out for children is helpful. Don't try to put a child to sleep at the peak of the waking cycle, or try to rouse the child at the peak of the sleepy cycle.

When giving or getting a good night back rub, plan it for about a half hour before the receiver's sleepy cycle peak. This way he or she will be awake to appreciate the start of the experience and begin to doze as the massage nears its end.

A CHILD'S SWEET DREAMS BACK RUB

In some families a child's recall of pleasant bedtime back rubs is a cherished memory. You can pass on relaxation techniques to your children as part of their legacy of knowing how to take care of their loved ones. A surprising number of parents I know have trained their children to give them back and foot rubs. Not only does this tradition help rejuvenate a tired parent but it also gives the child the reassuring feeling that he or she can contribute to taking care of the family in personal ways.

Perhaps you remember the wonderful, secure feeling of a bedtime back rub from a parent during your childhood. Give your child many of these loving experiences. No particular strokes are needed to give a good night massage. Simple, slow rubbing in circles covering most of the back is soothing. Rubbing the scalp is quieting. Long, smooth strokes from the shoulders to the lower back are particularly relaxing.

Allow your rhythms to get slower and slower as the massage progresses. You might want to give your child a good night kiss before the back rub rather than after so you don't startle them at the end of the sweet dreams strokes.

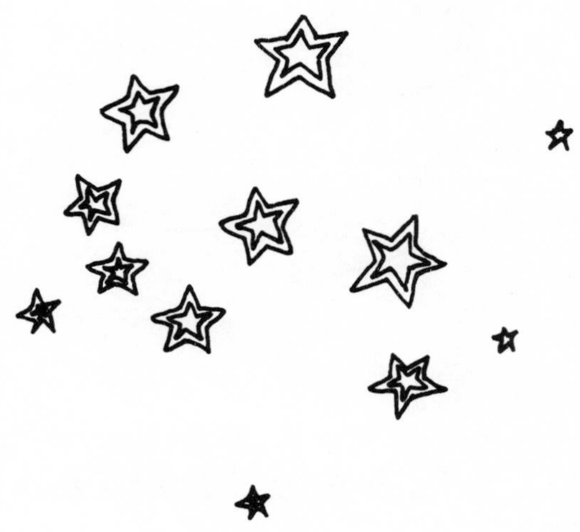

A Child's Sweet Dreams Back Rub

10 minutes

Circles—2 sets
Back Lift—1
Braiding—2
Palm Circles—6
Spine Sweep—8

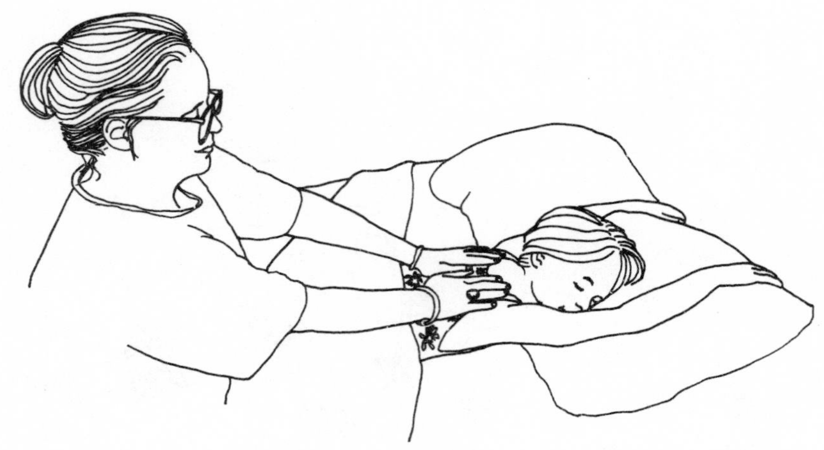

A CHILD'S SWEET DREAMS BACK RUB

Circles

Sit on the child's bed near his or her hips. If the child is lying on his or her stomach, place both your palms on the child's shoulders. Make slow circles with your hands moving away from each other from the spine toward the child's sides. Continue these circles down the back and up again.

Back Lift

If the child is lying on his or her back, you can lift the child slightly with little effort. Slide your hands under the child's middle back from opposite sides. Under the child, your fingertips should be on either side of the spine pointing toward each other. Press up with your fingertips into the groove

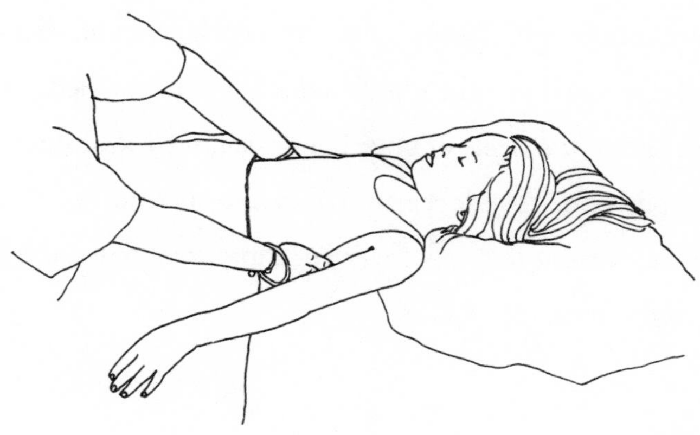

on either side of the spine. This action will raise the child's back slightly off the bed. If the child is sleepy and relaxed, he or she will give the weight over to your hands. The massage comes from the relaxed weight of the child's body pressing into your fingertips. Lower your fingertips and release the upward pressure. Move your hands down on the spine and repeat.

Braiding

Use the palms to do a motion like braiding hair. Begin with the heels of your hands resting on the bed to either side of the child's upper back. Move your fingertips toward each other, toward the spine. Just before they

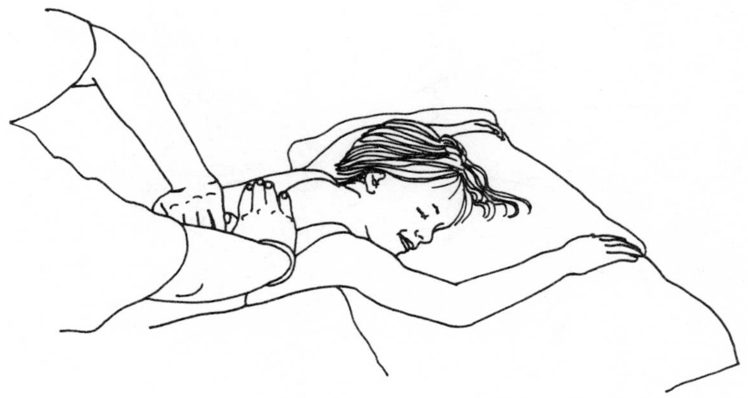

touch, move your hands slightly away from each other so that they can continue all the way down the child's sides again to the bed. Now reverse the motion: rotate the heels of your hands, sliding your fingertips back to the starting position. Your forearms will make an X as your hands pass over the spine. Repeat this crossover stroking up and down from the shoulders to the hips.

Palm Circles

Repeat the Palm Circles. This time do them only from the shoulders to the waist. This direction encourages rest by drawing the blood away from the heart. When your circles reach the waist, lift one palm and return it to the upper back. Then quickly bring your other hand to the shoulders also and begin the downward circles again.

Spine Sweep

Use this last stroke to connect all the others and give the child a sense of wholeness. Place your palms on your child's shoulders. Draw them along

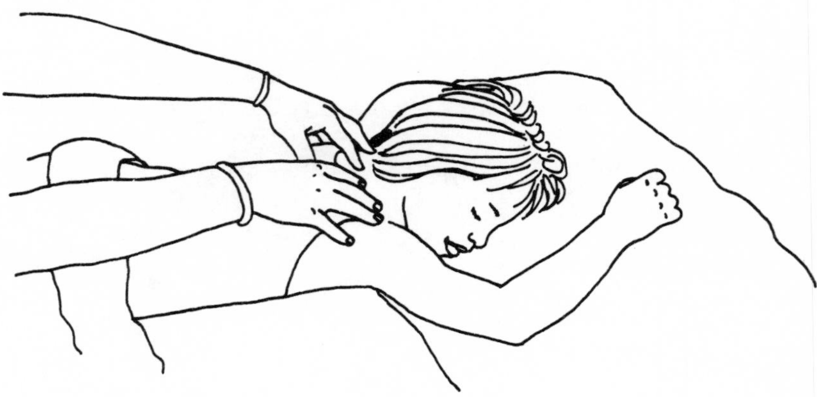

the muscles on either side of the spine down the back. When you reach the hips, angle your hands away from each other and lift them off the body. Make this a continuous, sweeping motion. Return your palms to the shoulders and start the sweep again with swift sweeps that become lighter each time you stroke.

GOOD NIGHT, SWEET FRIENDS & LOVERS

This is one performance for which the best bravo is your audience falling asleep. Everything you do is aimed at helping your friend go peacefully and deeply to sleep. Your strokes should be slow and smooth. Move from the shoulders down the back, encouraging the flow of blood away from the heart.

Positioning

Allow your friend to lie in the position he or she prefers for going to sleep so that no movement after the massage will be necessary. Whatever position they choose will afford you the chance to do a relaxing massage. Your friend may want to place pillows under the knees and calves if lying on the back, or between the knees if lying on the side. Raising the legs slightly relieves pressure on the lower back.

Stroking

Think of your strokes as slowing down your friend's metabolism, an aid to rest. Alternate specific area strokes with long, slow, sweeping strokes that cover the entire back. Moving from shoulders to lower back, your hands' pressure should get lighter and lighter as the massage progresses, until finally—when your hands leave the body at the end of the massage—they make no more sensation than that of a feather being blown off the back. Move quietly away from your sleeping friend.

Flights of Angels

When you fall asleep to the rhythms of a soothing back rub, the massage will work its gentle magic on your metabolism. Sleep well and wake up refreshed. Your back can be a doorway to your dreams.

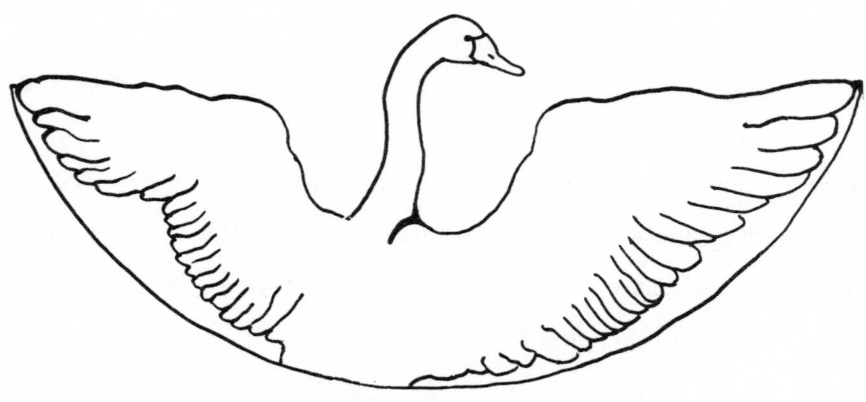

A Good Night Back Rub

15 minutes

Head Lift—1

Scalp Rub—whole scalp

Spine Lift—3

Neck Lift—1

Spine Drag—3

Upper Back & Neck Slide—3

Overlapping Palms—3

Spine Stretch—3

Spine Sweep—6

A GOOD NIGHT BACK RUB

The Good Night Back Rub can be done well with or without oils or nightclothes. The following strokes are done if your friend sleeps on his or her back or stomach. If your friend sleeps on his or her side, you can use the Pregnancy Back Rub strokes.

Head Lift

For this stroke your friend should be lying on her or his back. Using both hands, lift your friend's head as far forward as it will go. Move very

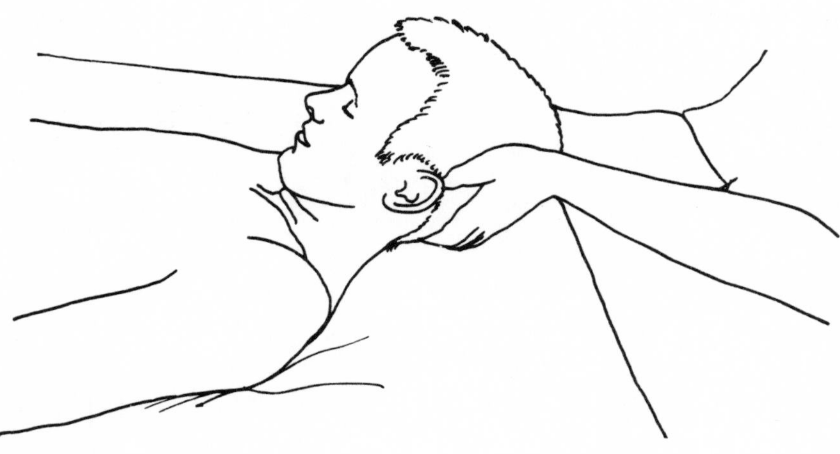

slowly. If you feel resistance, stop a moment and wait for your friend to relax the weight of the head into your hands. Then gently nudge the head a little forward. Don't ever push hard. The main point of this stroke is not to bend the neck but to allow your friend to give over the work of holding the head to you. Bring the head back down, moving very slowly to allow your friend to enjoy a vacation from holding the weight of his or her head.

Scalp Rub

Lift the head slightly and turn it to the right, supporting it in your right palm. Curl the fingers of your left hand and rub the scalp on the left side of the head with your fingertips. Moving your left hand in small circles, press hard enough that the skin moves a bit over the bone. Cover the entire side of the scalp with your circles. Repeat on the other side.

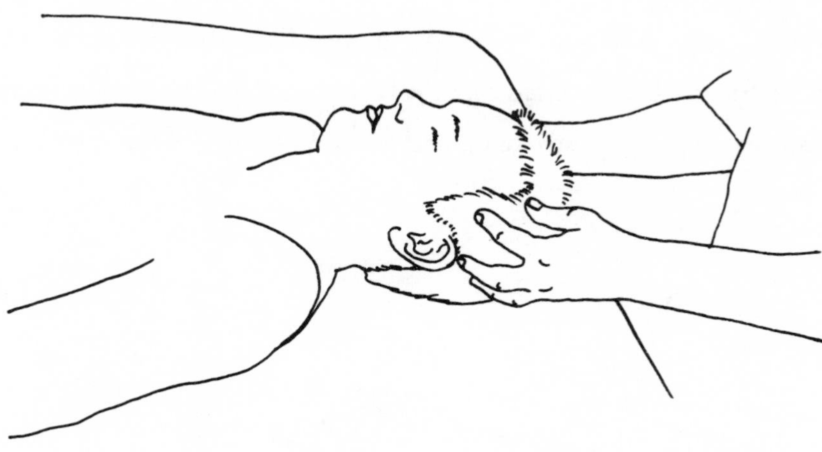

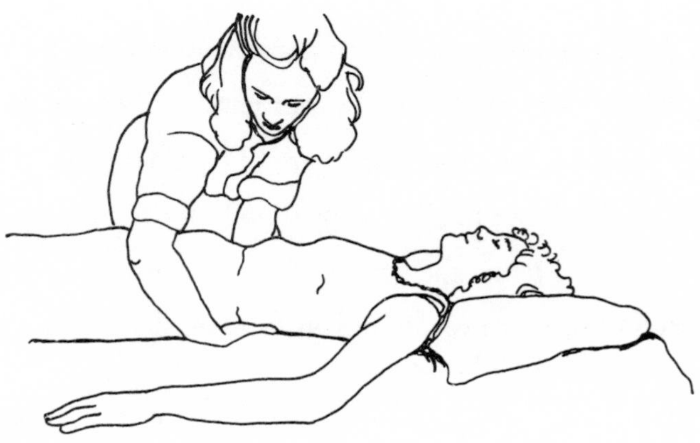

Spine Lift

Reach both hands palms up under either side of your friend's back at the waistline. Pointing toward each other, bring the fingertips to either side of the spine. Press the fingertips of both hands up and raise the middle of your friend's body a small distance off the bed. Hold for several seconds and release, lowering the back to the bed. Still pressing with the fingertips, slide your hands down a few inches and repeat. Being lifted will give your friend a special feeling of relaxation. If it is more comfortable to reach from one side of your friend, slide both hands, palms up, under the back on that side. With your fingertips on one side of the spine, press up so your friend's back is lifted slightly. Lower your fingers as your friend exhales. Repeat this stroke up and down both sides of the spine.

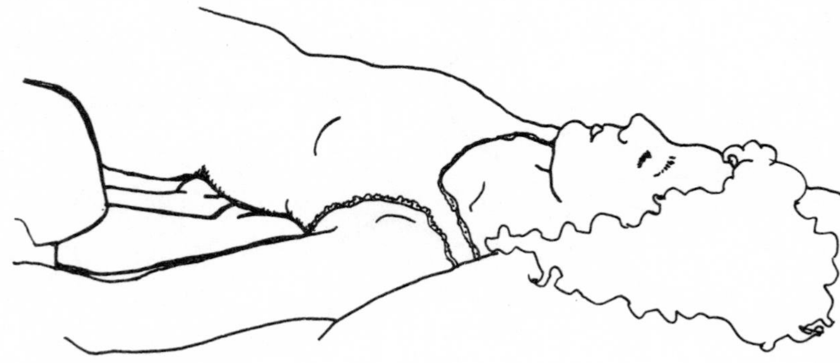

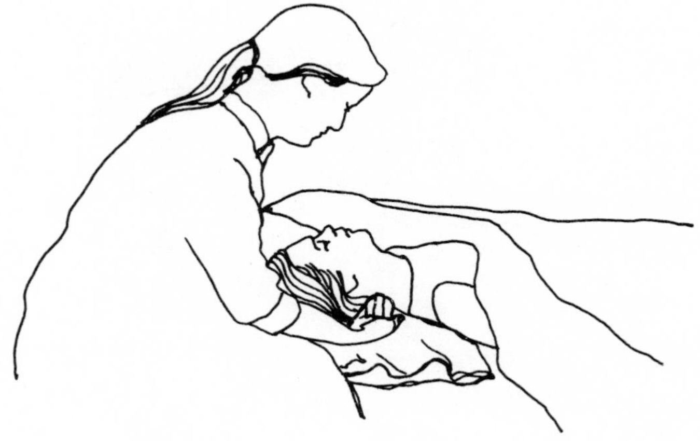

Neck Lift

This stroke is most easily done while you are standing or sitting above your friend's head or to one side. Slide whichever of your hands is stronger under your friend's neck. With your palm up, brace your hand on the bed and press upward into the neck muscles with your fingertips. Lift the neck a tiny bit while pressing and lower the head when releasing the pressure. Massage up and down the neck on the muscle to one side of the neck vertebrae. Then slide your fingers to the other side of the neck bones and repeat the stroke.

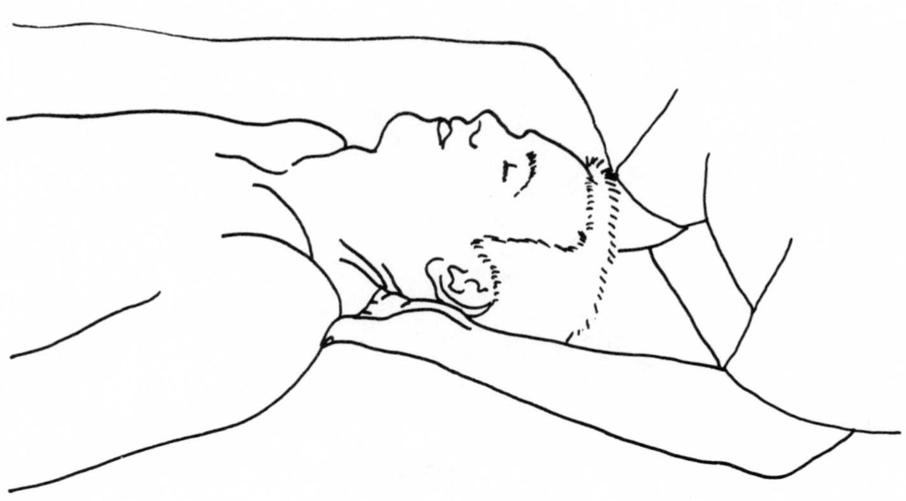

Spine Drag

For this stroke your friend should be lying on his or her back. Sitting above your friend's head, place both hands, palms up and fingers pointing toward the shoulders, on either side of the head. Without the help of your friend raising up, slide both hands under the upper back and push them as far down the back as you can. When you reach your limit, press your fingertips up on the grooves on either side of the spine. Now drag both hands back toward you pressing up as hard as you can. If your friend relaxes his or her weight onto your fingertips, this dragging creates a wonderful muscle relaxation. On the closing pulls, draw your fingertips up the back of the neck to the base of the skull.

Upper Back and Neck Slide

Slide your hands under the back of your friend's head and raise it slightly. Turn the head gently to the left until it rests in your left hand. Press the heel of your right hand onto the top of your friend's shoulder. Slide your cupped hand down the trapezius muscle to the tip of the shoulder. Circle your fingertips around the shoulder and onto the back. Move your fingers across the back toward the spine. Just before reaching the spine, pull your fingers onto the back of the neck. Continue up the neck until your fingertips reach the base of the skull. Then turn your hand so that your fingers

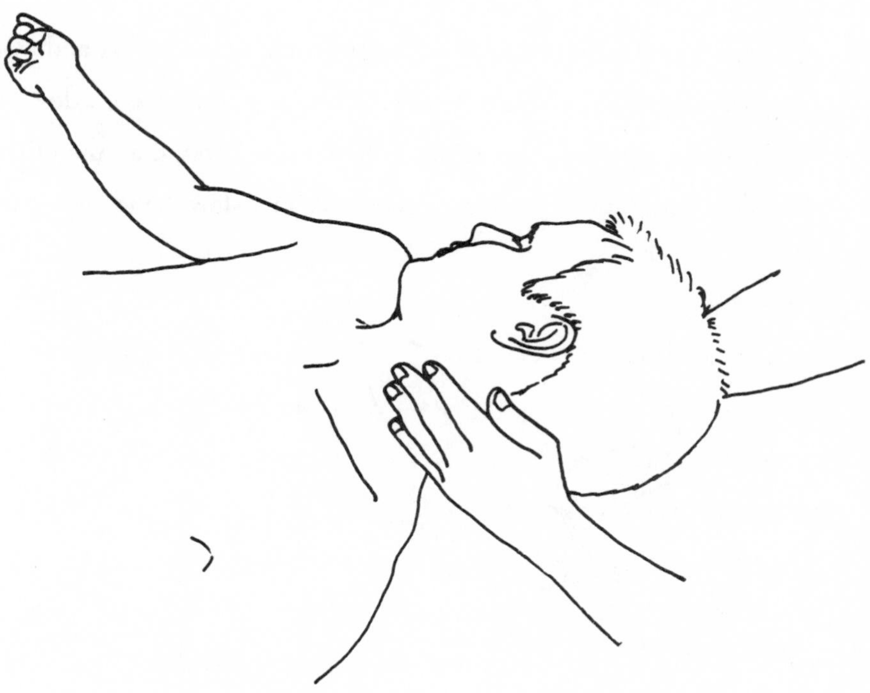

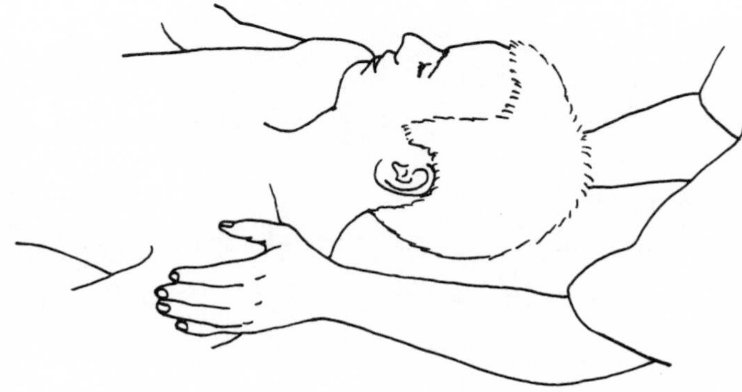

point up and you can glide them back down the side of the neck. From there you can continue to repeat the stroke several times.

Overlapping Palms

If your friend is lying on his or her stomach, reach across and work on the side opposite you. Start just below the armpit and work down the side to the waist, then back up again. Pull first one hand, then the other, up from the bed, fingers pointing downward, in a slow, hand-over-hand

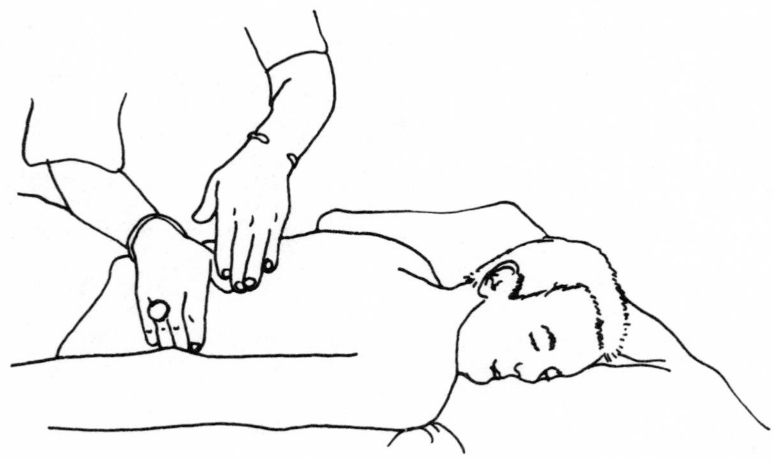

rhythm. Each pull begins just as the previous one is about to end. Work several times up and then down both sides of the torso, moving to your friend's other side as needed.

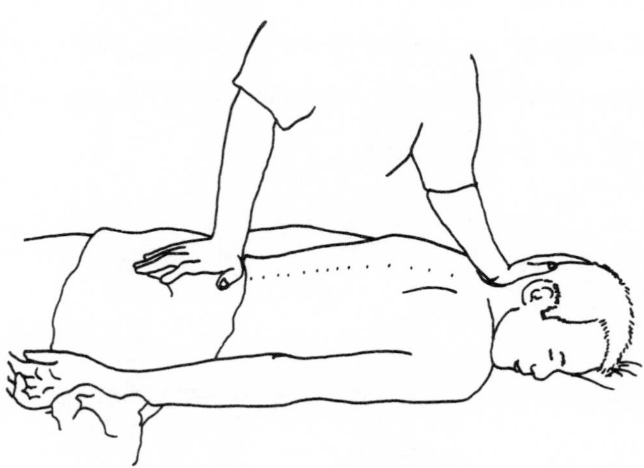

Spine Stretch

While lying facedown, your friend's head should be facing away from you to the left. Standing to your friend's right side, take the heel of your right hand and lodge it under your friend's occipital ridge (the base of the skull). Take the heel of your left hand and place it on the sacrum (the triangular bone at the base of the spine), with your fingertips pointing toward the left hip. Gently and gradually apply pressure to the heels of both hands, moving them very slightly outward so that you are stretching your friend's spine from top to bottom, by pressing the head up and the sacrum down. Release the pressure gradually.

Spine Sweep

Place your palms on your friend's shoulders. Draw them along the muscles on either side of the spine, down the back and over the hips. As you cross the hips, angle your hands away from each other and lift them off the body. Return your palms to the shoulders and begin the sweep again with light, swift strokes. Make the pace of this stroke slower each time you repeat it. A soothing back rub relaxes the giver as well as the receiver. You'll sleep better too. Sweet dreams.

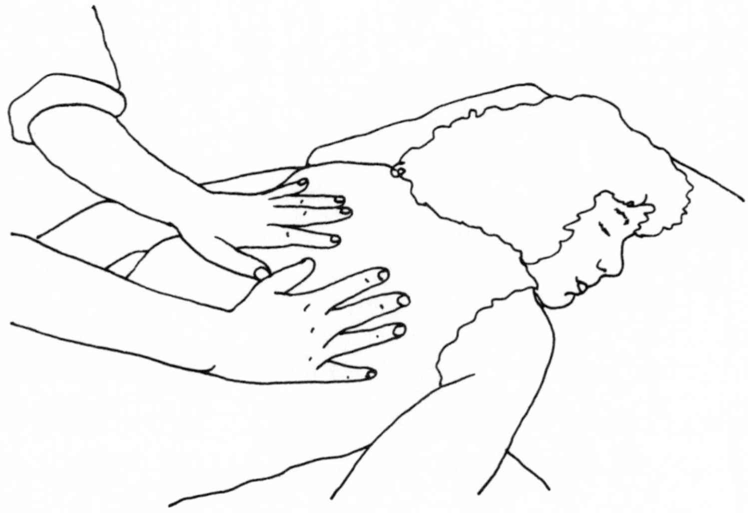

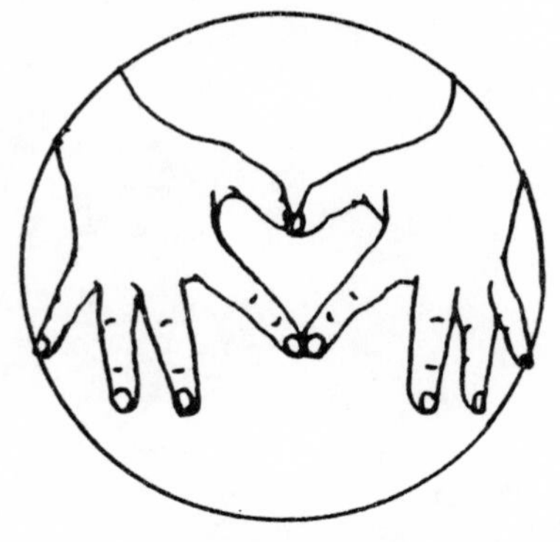

DESIGNING YOUR OWN BACK RUBS

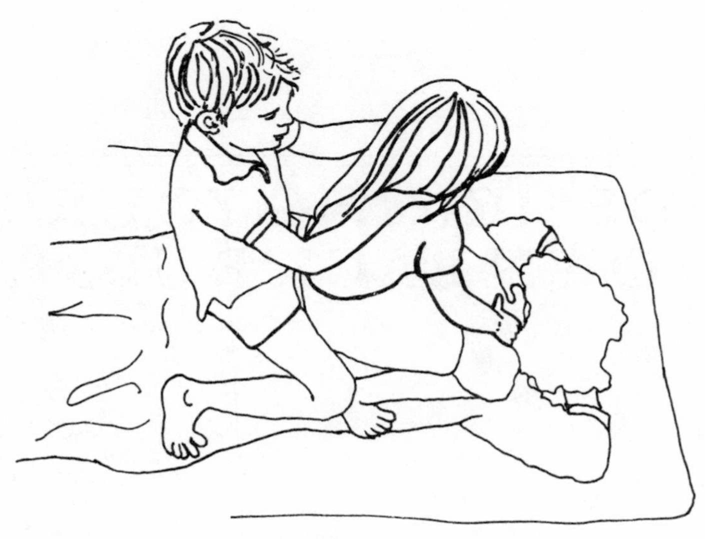

PRIVATE LABEL BACK RUBS

The back rubs in this book can be used on any occasion. You can combine several of the short ones to produce longer, more luxurious massages.

You can change the sequence of strokes within a back rub, and it will feel like a new one to the receiver. Or you can put together single strokes from various back rubs in your own sequence to make a new back rub.

Eureka!

You may even want to invent your own strokes. This can happen haphazardly. While giving a back rub, you may accidentally do something new that's worth repeating. When you make a transition move to connect two strokes, you may discover that this pattern makes a nice stroke on its own. Also you may have a feel for the medium and find that making up your own strokes is fun. The basic strokes of popular massage have become old standards because many people like them, and these strokes take care of

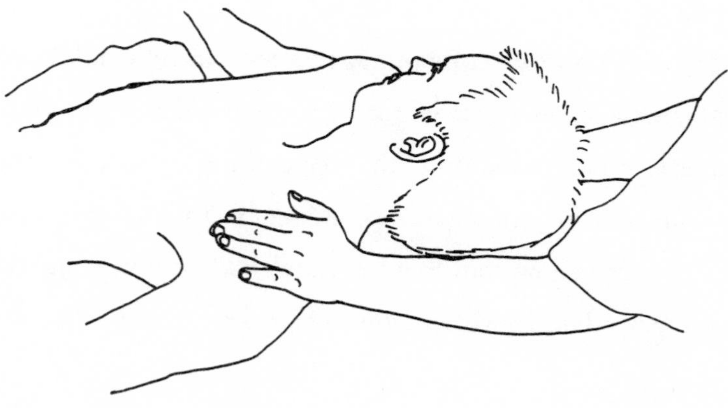

the major muscle groups. However, new strokes keep your massages exciting, keep you from being bored, and generally delight the receiver. Pointers on stroke construction and invention follow.

DESIGNING STROKES

Doing is inspiring. Your hands naturally invent motion patterns if you relax and let them. Listen to your impulses and experiment. Receiving is also inspiring, because you feel glitches or missing links as the receiver of the massage and can easily imagine what would feel better.

Combine and reverse. Often combining two strokes as a unit can work well. Combined strokes feel different to the receiver because the transition action is new and because together, strokes cover a larger area and give the receiver a different awareness of the body. For instance, receiving a circular stroke at the base of your neck and then a circular stroke on your lower back gives a very different sensation than having both areas massaged simultaneously.

A muscle or body contour calls out for its own individual treatment. As you massage the shoulder blade, for instance, you'll find that your hand naturally tends to mold itself around the shape of the bone, and certain movements with your fingers are more comfortable to do in this area than others. See if you can allow your mind to wander while continuing the back rub; you may come up with interesting strokes. It's a bit like absentmindedly circling the rim of a glass with your forefinger. When unchecked, your hands usually find the contours of what they're touching and define its shape rhythmically.

Think about the function as well as the shape of a body part. It will inspire you to invent strokes that complement the muscle's natural movement. Learning some anatomy can help you think of more strokes also.

Be silly. With the consent of the receiver, try massaging with rhythms and kinds of strokes and patterns that you normally would consider silly or awkward. Move your hands in new ways even if doing so seems odd at first. This approach will help you find ways of moving that you otherwise wouldn't try. Some of these may turn out to be great. An off-the-wall R & D session also reminds you that massage is basically fun. And the spirit of the play may help you invent some joyous strokes.

Listen to the feedback and ideas for new strokes you get from the person you're massaging. Try them out. What feels good to one may feel good to many.

Try a stroke you learned for one area on another. See if with alterations a stroke will suit a new area. Try massaging with a part of your hand you've not used before, such as your fists for long, smooth strokes or your forearms for spreading motions.

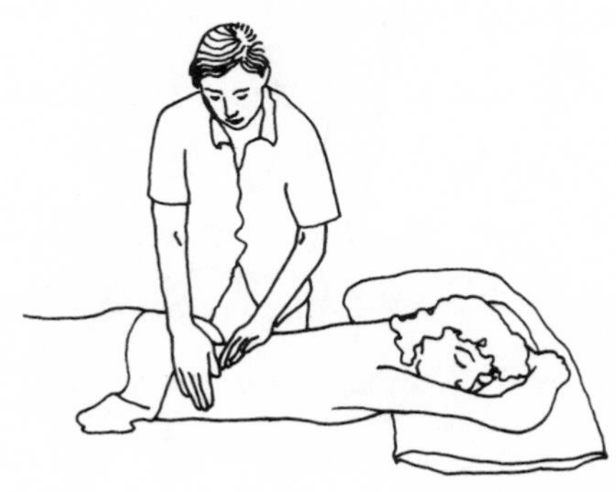

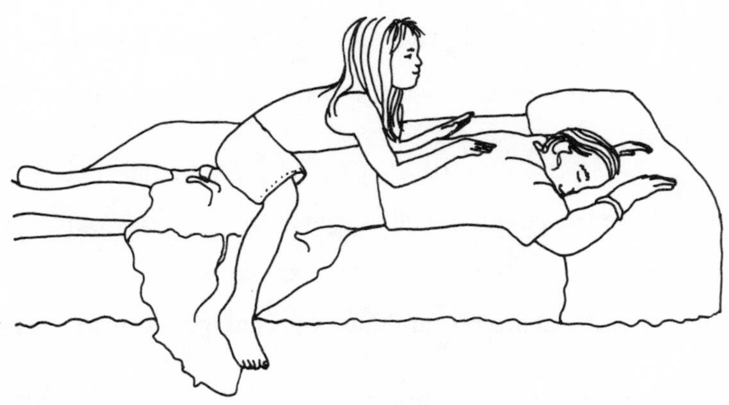

Name your inventions. Names help you remember a stroke and distinguish it from another. Credit co-authors. I showed an exercise I'd invented to a friend, and he said I looked like a hard-boiled egg rolling around in a pan while doing it. I named it Charlie's Egg Roll. He was pleased, and I'll never forget it. You can also experiment with working backward in this process by thinking of a name and then trying to invent a stroke that fits it. This may help you create a new motion that feels good.

Close your eyes. Giving a massage with your eyes closed is a fine way to increase the level of "thinking with your hands." You will be guided by touch rather than sight and be more likely to invent something that feels great.

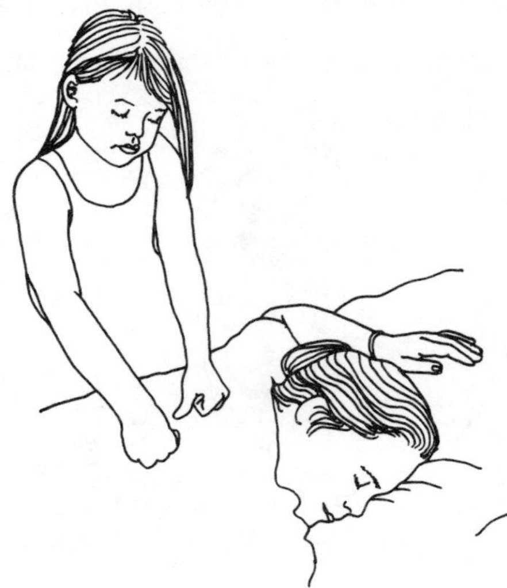

DESIGNING WHOLE MASSAGES

Here are some guidelines to help you structure a complete massage:

Start slow and **work up to speedy** strokes.

Start with grand-scale strokes and **work toward details** on smaller areas.

Make your transitions between strokes gradual so the receiver experiences the whole massage as a continuous stroke.

Start light and **work up to heavier** pressure.

If you lift a limb for a stroke, only move it gently in its natural direction.

Slow down as you near the close of the massage.

Do some grand finale strokes that cover large areas — even the whole body — to close. This leaves your friend with a sense of connected wholeness.

Learn from feedback. Requests can be the mother of invention. Do only what feels good to your friend.

Have fun tailoring the conditions of the back rub to your friend's and your desires.

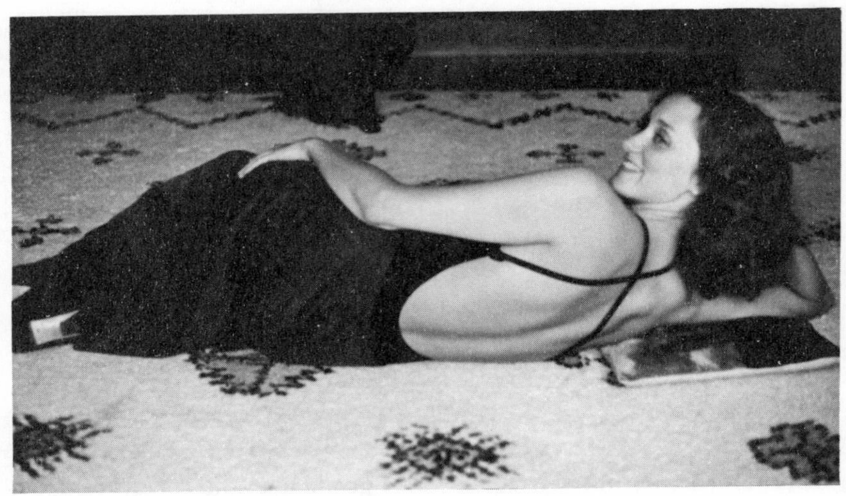

About the Author

Anne Kent Rush was born in Mobile, Alabama. She is a descendant of Dr. Benjamin Rush, an American health revolutionary who signed the Declaration of Independence. Rush is the author of *Getting Clear: Body Work for Women; Moon, Moon;* and *The Basic Back Book*; co-author of *Feminism as Therapy;* and illustrator and editor of *The Massage Book*.

Anne Kent Rush was on the training staffs of Alyssum Center and of Esalen Institute in California. She was a partner in Moon Books. Now she produces a series of children's travel books on wildlife conservation. The first in the series is *Greta Bear Goes to Yellowstone National Park*. Rush currently resides in the Shenandoah Valley, West Virginia. She continues her research and writing on health and is working on a novel set in China.